# Fat Loss Habits

*I would like to dedicate this book to my wife. Without her believing in me, I wouldn't have had the confidence to start writing in the first place.*

# Fat Loss Habits

**Ben Carpenter**

balance

New York   Boston

Balance
Hachette Book Group
1290 Avenue of the Americas
New York, NY 10104
GCP-Balance.com
@GCPBalance

First published in 2025 in Great Britain by Short Books, an imprint of Octopus Publishing Group Ltd., a Hachette UK Company

First Balance edition: January 2025

Balance is an imprint of Grand Central Publishing. The Balance name and logo are registered trademarks of Hachette Book Group, Inc.

The publisher is not responsible for websites (or their content) that are not owned by the publisher.

The Hachette Speakers Bureau provides a wide range of authors for speaking events. To find out more, go to hachettespeakersbureau.com or email HachetteSpeakers@hbgusa.com.

Balance books may be purchased in bulk for business, educational, or promotional use. For information, please contact your local bookseller or the Hachette Book Group Special Markets Department at special.markets@hbgusa.com.

LCCN: 2024949503

ISBNs: 9781538768655 (trade paperback); 9781538768662 (ebook)

Printed in the United States of America

LSC-C

Printing 1, 2024

# Contents

# Note on the US Edition

To my American friends,

Although I am fortunate enough to also live in America now, this project originated with a publisher in England, where I lived for the majority of my life. As such, some of the words, phrases, and measurements included within will be more familiar to English readers than to you—but I use plenty of US-flavored language and data, too. I have tried my best to include explanations and parenthetical notes to translate anything that you might be less familiar with, but some graphs from research studies use metric (like grams and kilograms) rather than imperial measurements (like ounces and pounds). This was out of my control; due to copyright restrictions, we're only allowed to use images from scientific sources if we keep certain ones as is rather than reformat them. If you stumble across any of these, know this is not due to a lack of love or consideration from me or my publishing teams.

# You Don't Need Another Diet

Every New Year, gyms across the world experience an influx of new members. If you went into your local fitness center and asked them what their busiest months are, I would bet my lunch money that they would say the beginning of each year is when they see the highest membership spike; a wave of enthusiastic people sign up, pay their membership fees and start their New Year's resolutions.

Unfortunately, it is also no secret that this excitement tends to wear off quickly and, by the end of the year, most of those new members will never set foot in that gym again. Although fitness clubs like to be secretive about this fact and do not like to gloat about how many of their paying members don't even visit anymore, by some estimates, over 60 percent of members fail to exercise regularly for the full first 12 months of their membership, according to one research study in Norway.[1] This is great for gyms that make money from people not even using the facilities, but far from ideal for the customers who have abandoned their fitness ambitions so swiftly. Other research paints an even worse picture. A study in Brazil revealed that over 60 percent of members leave the gym within the first three months, and a smidge less than a measly 4 percent of them stick it out for more than the first year.[2] Why do you think so many gyms tie you into a 12-month-minimum membership? Because they make a large chunk of their money from those of you who sign up but stop using the facilities. If all of their members actually went to the gym consistently, the place would be too overcrowded to use. Their business model literally relies on charging people who don't go anymore.

Now, take this knowledge and apply it to dieting. How many times have you wanted to lose body fat, so you started a diet, followed it for a little while, then decided to throw in the towel and go back to what you were doing before? Maybe you got bored of the diet. Maybe you struggled to follow it because it was too difficult. Maybe you are one of the many people who just realized that dieting is not fun, and that avoiding your favorite foods might have worked for a short while, but soon your rate of weight loss was surpassed by how quickly you lost the will to live. In Western countries like America, every single year, nearly *half* of all adults try to lose weight at least once,[3] and high dieting rates like this are common around the globe,[4] which is a telltale sign of a really big problem.

Diets don't work. At least, not in the way that people commonly approach them.

Just as people join the gym, stop going over time and then join again later down the line, this loop is also indicative of common dieting practices. Many new gym members report a pattern of weight cycling—otherwise known as yo-yo dieting—and trying to lose weight using unhealthy strategies.[5] Ultimately, too many people are caught in the trap of aggressively crash dieting, losing weight temporarily and repeating this yo-yo cycle year after year. This book is for those of you who are fed up with this and want to change.

If I told you that I wanted to retire wealthy, and that I planned on cramming in as much overtime as possible for a few weeks before quitting my job out of exhaustion, would you tell me that this was a sensible idea? No. You would tell me that it made zero sense in comparison to having a long-term earning and saving strategy.

If I told you that I wanted to learn to play the guitar, and that my plan was to practice every hour of the day until my fingertips became bloodied and I had to stop after a couple of weeks, would you tell me that this was smart? Obviously not. You would tell me that, if I wanted to get really good on the guitar, I would need to practice consistently for many years rather than in an intense burst for a short period of time. And if I wanted to be good on the guitar for the rest of my life, I would need to make sure I kept practicing in some capacity forevermore, not just for a few weeks.

If I told you that I wanted to be fit, strong and athletic when I was elderly, so I could play with my grandchildren and hopefully be the healthiest person in the nursing home, would you tell me to work out and diet intensely for three months, only to quit the gym because I was sick of it? Also no.

Instinctively, we know that, if we have a long-term goal, it makes no sense to approach that goal with habits that we can only maintain for a short period of time, right? So, why are so many people in the weight loss industry focused on ramming brand-new, unsustainable diets down our throats every year, instead of offering us a solution that lasts?

Unless your goal is to follow an overly restrictive diet and lose body fat briefly before regaining that lost fat and repeating the cycle over and over again, let's zoom out and take a look at the bigger, more important picture.

If you want lasting success, I hope you know that you don't need yet another short-term crash diet, another unnecessarily rigid meal plan or another fat loss fad that is popular now but nobody will be talking about in ten years' time. So, what do you need instead? You need to be brought up-to-date on the newest science on long-term weight management and learn how to implement healthy habits—behaviors that you can actually sustain over a longer period of time. My goal in this book is to help you get better results for less effort by exploring 13 healthy habits and letting you choose what works best for you, then assist you in turning those habits into something that becomes second nature to you.

So, let's shift your focus toward what really matters. This is *Fat Loss Habits*.

# 1

# Addressing the Real Problem

Before we get to the healthy habits that can help you achieve sustained fat loss, which we'll explore in Chapter 5, we need to address the factors that derail us and stop us realizing our long-term fat loss goals. I entered the fitness industry as a young, oily-faced teenager who loved exercise so much I asked if I could help out at my local gym. I wasn't qualified in anything, and I didn't care what I did there, I just knew it was the career path I wanted to embark on. I started off by answering the phone, cleaning the equipment and just making sure nobody accidentally injured themselves by using the machines incorrectly. Then I trained as a personal trainer back in 2006, which means my entire adult life has been spent working in the fitness industry. I have had the pleasure of spending thousands of hours not just working face-to-face with people like you, but also communicating with them on social media. So, you can trust me when I say I have talked to more people about their health and fitness goals than almost anyone else on the planet. This puts me in a fortunate enough position to see some common themes and trends.

Out of all the clients who come to me asking for help, what do you think their number one goal is? To lose body fat. It isn't even a close call. Sure, a lot of people want to get stronger, fitter and healthier in general, and a small subsection of people have niche goals like wanting to get more agile for their pole dancing job or wanting to train their neck so they are less likely to be knocked unconscious when they are playing rugby (both real examples), but by an absolute mile, fat loss is the most requested goal.

This shouldn't be a massive surprise. After all, many people feel like they are struggling with their weight. Perhaps what is more of a surprise is that, for people who weigh more, just the act of managing their weight is often seen as a higher priority than super important goals like improving their health, fitness and well-being.[1]

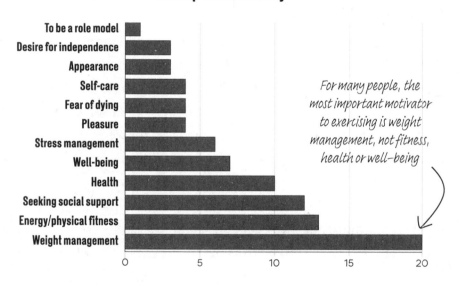

**Importance Scores of Motives Toward Physical Activity in People with Obesity[2]**

For many people, the most important motivator to exercising is weight management, not fitness, health or well-being

The reasons behind this are complex. Although many people do want to diet because they think it will improve their health, the larger motivators are often appearance and self-esteem.[3] Unfortunately, this can also be driven by more negative outside influences, like social pressure from friends and family or because they have faced weight discrimination.[4] People think that perhaps if they are thinner, they will be seen as more attractive to others or feel more comfortable in their own skin. Commonly, they give explanations like having a holiday coming up and worrying about feeling embarrassed on the beach, or being newly single, and feeling that being thinner will increase their chances of finding a new partner, which actually says a lot about how they think other people will treat them rather than how they feel about themselves.

## A Growing Trend

If you have found yourself getting heavier over time, or you feel self-conscious about your weight, rest assured that you are not alone. In the past 50 years or so there has been a general trend for the global population to weigh more than it used to, and this is seen across age and sex demographics. Between 1975 and 2016, the number of people with obesity across the world was estimated to have increased from 5 million to 50 million for girls, 6 million to 74 million for boys, 69 million to 390 million for women, and 31 million to 281 million for men.[5] Although there is obviously some variance, this trend is essentially seen across most countries.

This "obesity epidemic" is a hot topic, as there are many health risks associated with having higher levels of body fat. These include cardiovascular disease[6] and heart failure,[7] several different types of cancer,[8] type 2 diabetes,[9] knee osteoarthritis,[10] reduced quality of life,[11] and a higher risk of all-cause mortality.[12] In simple terms, if you gain a lot of weight from where you are now, you might notice certain aspects of your health declining. This doesn't mean that everyone who weighs less is definitely healthier than everyone who weighs more, or that some people weigh more without noticing any adverse health effects, or that people who weigh more deserve to be bullied, which are some of the common narratives you might hear about people in larger bodies. It just means that the risk of some health conditions can be elevated if you gain a lot of weight, and some health conditions can be improved when some people lose weight.

Now, here is the funny thing that I don't think a lot of people realize. Despite the fact that, globally, people have been gaining weight, the percentage of people who are actively trying to lose weight also looks like it has been going up, not down. For example, using some estimates from America, around 7 percent of men and 14 percent of women reported trying to lose weight between 1950 and 1966.[13] By the late 1980s this had increased to around 24 percent of men and 39 percent of women.[14,15] This continued to go up between 1999 and 2016, when the percentage of all American adults who reported trying to lose weight grew again, from 34 to 42 percent.[16] Using the latest numbers available, the Centers for Disease Control and Prevention (CDC), the national public health agency in the US, claims that nearly half of all adults and nearly 40 percent of all adolescents tried to lose weight in the last year, and these rates were even higher among women and girls.[17,18] People often mistakenly associate weight gain with a lack of willpower, but if our whole society really was lazy and lacked willpower, this would be reflected in an absence of dieting, not an increase. If more people are proactively trying to lose weight than ever, this doesn't suggest we just stopped giving a shit, does it? Clearly, something bigger is at play here. As society has been gaining weight, it makes sense that more people try to lose weight in response to that, right? But the growing "obesity epidemic" that people keep warning us about is direct evidence that the increase in dieting is not fixing the real problem, it's more like throwing a cup of water onto a forest fire.

### Prevalence of Obesity (BMI ≥30 kg/m²) Between 1975 and 2016 According to Geographical Region[19] (Data shown for females ≥20 years of age)

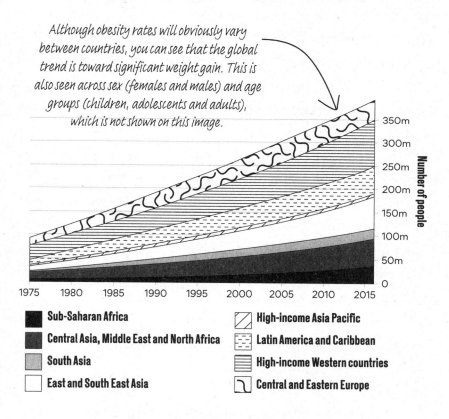

Although obesity rates will obviously vary between countries, you can see that the global trend is toward significant weight gain. This is also seen across sex (females and males) and age groups (children, adolescents and adults), which is not shown on this image.

Number of people

| | |
|---|---|
| ■ Sub-Saharan Africa | ▨ High-income Asia Pacific |
| ■ Central Asia, Middle East and North Africa | ▦ Latin America and Caribbean |
| ▨ South Asia | ▤ High-income Western countries |
| □ East and South East Asia | ⌐ Central and Eastern Europe |

This teaches us a super important lesson—and let me give you a parallel example to explain the issue. Imagine you were in charge of a whole country, and you heard that the rate of homelessness was going up. Obviously, because you are (hopefully) a caring person, you want to fix the problem, so you need to work out a strategy to take care of people. To kick things off, your adviser tells you that you need to tell everyone without a home that they need to work harder to find one. It kind of makes sense on paper, so you go with it. After a while, you notice that the rate of homelessness is continuing to rise, but you also find out that the number of people who are proactively trying to find a home is also rising. You realize that this strategy is not working, so you start to ask yourself what is really causing the dilemma. Is there a cost-of-living crisis? Has the economy fallen to shit? Is there a shortage of available homes? Is there a lack of jobs for people to work in so they can't afford the money to pay rent? These are the real factors that are causing the issue.

So, if more and more people are slowly gaining weight over time despite a higher percentage of them actively trying to lose weight, we need to stop and consider what the driving forces are. It's not just you as an individual, it's a much bigger systemic issue that is occurring behind the scenes. The "obesity epidemic" is so rampant that many researchers rack their brains trying to figure out just how many factors are causing people to gain weight.[20,21,22] In fact, it is such a complex problem that it is surprisingly difficult to pinpoint the exact triggers that are driving this global trend,[23] but let's discuss some of the biggest culprits.

## What's Really Causing the Obesity Epidemic?

If you wanted to gain as much weight as possible in the shortest period of time, what would you do? The answer is obvious, isn't it? You would eat as much food and do as little exercise as possible. At its core, weight gain is a very simple mismatch between the amount of energy you consume and how much you burn. If you want to lose weight, you are told to eat less food and be more active.

Sounds simple, right? So, the million-dollar question is: Why do so many people find it so fucking difficult to do?

## Sedentary lifestyles

Let's rewind 70 years or so, prior to the sharpest rise in body weights across the world largely agreed upon to have started in the 1970s. Consider what your life might have been like compared to today. Back then, there was far less technology, so you wouldn't have spent your day in the office working at a computer or working from your comfortable home with a laptop in front of you. Televisions weren't as common as they are now and you definitely wouldn't have had the luxury of hundreds of channels and thousands of shows and movies available at your fingertips, so the likelihood of you wanting to spend your evenings binge-watching your favorite program was slim to none. Especially because remote controls weren't even a thing then. Nowadays, the idea of having to get up to press a button on the TV every time you want to change the channel sounds absurd and would absolutely interrupt the mindless doomscrolling tendencies that streaming platforms love you to have. Game consoles were yet to exist, so the concept of children being immersed in screens at home was unheard of. The prospect of kids playing their favorite video games on the move, on phones or tablets, was not even within the realm of possibility. These days, technology has the ability to entertain us, but a lot of that entertainment encourages us to be sedentary.

Technology can also make our lives easier. We have more access to cars and public transport, which save us from walking as much as we used to. We have escalators and elevators that spare us the effort of climbing staircases. We have the internet to help us buy whatever we fancy without ever having to walk around the shops. We have washing machines and dishwashers to clean our clothes and dishes at the touch of a button, which relieves us from doing them by hand. We don't even really need to exert energy to brush our teeth anymore. Many of us just hold the brush in our mouths and let the vibrations from the electric toothbrush work their magic.

Once upon a time, if you wanted to stay alive, you would need to go out hunting and foraging for your own food, which you would then perhaps patiently cook over a fire that you had built yourself. It's a shitload of work for one meal, right? Nowadays, even though we have local shops that conveniently stock everything we want, we don't even need to leave our homes if we aren't in the mood. Just a few taps on our laptops and someone can bring that food right to our doors. It's not that we are getting lazier as such, it's more that we are using technology to our advantage to save us time and energy. If a company offers home delivery, it allows us to do something else with the time we would have spent shopping; like doing more work, or playing with our kids, or just chilling out because we are tired after a long day.

Many of us have spent years, or even decades, of our lives waking up, hopping in the car to drive to work, and getting in an elevator to take us up to our office, where we spend the next eight hours sitting at a desk before getting back in that elevator, driving home and spending the rest of the evening sitting on the couch. Generally speaking, our overall environment is dictating that we exert less energy in our daily lives than ever before, so should we be surprised that many of us aren't as active as we would like to be? To write this book, I will have spent the majority of my days in front of my laptop for well over a year. Sometimes I have to force myself to leave the house because the step counter on my smartwatch subtly reminds me that I am turning into a recluse who spends 95 percent of his life barely moving. It doesn't mean I am lazy. It just means this is what I do for work, you know?

The point is, if moving less is one surefire contributor to gaining weight, we have absolutely nailed this as an art form. The trend toward physical inactivity is thought to be one of the primary reasons why our society weighs more than it used to.[24,25,26,27] I don't know about you, but the only way I could physically move less during my workday is if I just took my laptop to bed with me and wrote this book there instead.

### Fast-food access

Of course, the other part of the equation is eating more, and it's probably no surprise that what we eat nowadays has also changed a smidge. That's obviously underselling it—how we eat today is a bazillion miles away from how we used to eat, for so many different reasons it's impossible to quantify them all. As an example, let's imagine you are a child born today and compare your environment to a child's born one hundred years ago.

First, you will grow up surrounded by more fast-food outlets than at any other point in history. The first ever McDonald's opened in 1955 and, at the time of writing, they now report to own over 38,000 outlets in more than one hundred countries.[28] The first ever Kentucky Fried Chicken opened in 1952 and they currently claim to own over 25,000 restaurants spanning more than 145 countries.[29] Similar stories can be seen elsewhere, with Pizza Hut and Burger King both owning approximately 19,000 restaurants each.[30,31] This is just one solid indicator of how much our overall nutrition landscape has changed. If you were born one hundred years ago, you wouldn't have been surrounded by this abundance of high-calorie, deep-fried, high-sugar, super-convenient and designed to be as delicious as possible fast food. Given that just four of the top fast-food chains own over 100,000 outlets and are worth hundreds of billions of dollars, collectively, it's fair to say they are a growing and highly influential contributor to our food supply.

As fast-food and "quick-service" restaurants have become more commonplace, it isn't surprising that more of us are lured in with the convenience of having food served in an instant. After all, if we have a busy day at work, we can nip into a fast-food outlet on our lunch break, have a tasty meal and be done in less time than it would take for us to make that meal from scratch. Using America as a specific example, in 1978 it was estimated that 82 percent of the average diet was food prepared at home, but over 20 years this dropped to 68 percent as people started eating more restaurant and take-out food. In 1978, 4 percent of the average adult's diet came from fast-food restaurants specifically and this tripled to 12 percent in the same mere 20-year period.[32] As fast-food outlets grew in popularity, they expanded their menus to do their best to lure you in with a wider selection of tasty dishes, and many of these dishes tended to be bigger and more calorie-dense than they were previously.[33] Research studies have analyzed portion sizes at fast-food restaurants plus those of some popular ultra-processed food brands, like chocolate and soda drinks, and found that some foods are now five times bigger than when they were first introduced.[34] In the 1970s, brands started offering significantly more large portions of foods that exceeded government recommendations, suggesting that the food you buy nowadays is probably significantly bigger than if you had bought the equivalent 50 or more years ago.[35]

## Portion Size Availability in the US Marketplace: Comparing Products When First Launched to 2021[36]

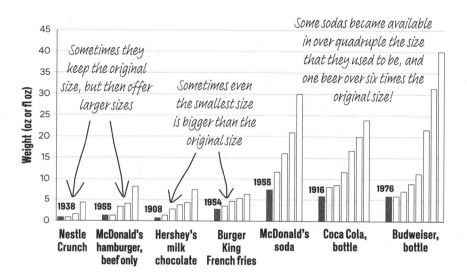

By some recent estimates, over half of all American adults eat food from standard and quick-service restaurants every single day, and fast-food options specifically comprise approximately 37 percent of their total daily calorie intake.[37] Fast-food outlets tend to be more prevalent in poorer areas and less common in wealthy areas,[38] meaning that calorie-dense fast food is likely to be a more attractive proposition for those on lower incomes. After all, if you gave your teenage child $5 to grab some lunch, they could buy a tasty cheeseburger, fries and a soda and still come home with some change, so why would they go next door to the fancy health food cafe that charges more money for a boring yet ridiculously expensive salad?

In my opinion, it's not surprising that we eat more fast food than we used to when that food is often cheaper, created to be tastier thanks to added fat, sugar, salt and flavorings, and more convenient than most other options. Blaming people for eating fast food is a bit like putting a delicious-looking cake in front of a hungry person and then telling them off for eating it. If we grow up surrounded by fast-food restaurants, let's not act shocked if we choose to eat that fast food.

### The evolution of convenience foods

Of course, it's not just fast-food meals that are more common. There is also a growing abundance of high-calorie snack foods. These are sometimes referred to as "discretionary foods," the kinds of things you would not consider your core meals, often high in sugar, fat and calories, and not recommended to be a large portion of your diet.[39] When you are in the mood for something to nibble on but you aren't ready to stop working to grab a proper meal, what do you eat? Well, don't worry, because you are surrounded by options here too.

When you put petrol (that's gas, for our American friends) in your car and you go in to pay for it, what is normally at the counter? A selection of chocolate bars and candies to tempt you into the upsell, adding something small to your fuel purchase so you give them more of your money. If you are walking along a city street you will often see doughnut shops, kiosks selling cookies, and cafes with some beautiful cakes and pastries sitting in the window, doing their best to catch your attention. These discretionary foods tend to be convenient, delicious and not particularly nutritious.

Although they are increasingly common, it is actually very difficult to study the impact of all of them combined because you can't exactly measure every source of discretionary snacks in an entire city. That would be harder than counting grains of sand on a beach in the middle of a hurricane. What you can do is pick one type of outlet and zoom in on it, so let's discuss vending machines, specifically. Although they are not exactly new, what is new is how prevalent they are. If you walk through an airport, train station, bus station, university campus, school or work cafeteria, chances are you will see at least one vending machine. These have come under scrutiny for creating an obesogenic environment, which is a fancy term for "this probably nudges people toward gaining weight."[40] This is because vending machines tend to be filled with calorie-dense mouthgasmic discretionary snacks that are easy to get when you are on the go. Although you might see the occasional more nutritious vending machine, these are far from common. Fresh and nutritious food doesn't tend to work super well in vending machines, for obvious reasons. Can you imagine what would happen to a machine full of ready-to-eat salads and freshly prepared fruit? The food inside would start going bad unless it was regularly emptied and restocked, which costs a business money. Seeing a rotten apple or moldy salad behind the glass would hardly make you want to put your coins into the machine, would it? Thankfully, chocolate bars, chips and candy are here to save the day with their long shelf lives, as they require minimal machine maintenance. According to one previous analysis of American schools, the most common items found in vending machines were chips (referred to as crisps in other countries), crackers, cakes, cookies, toaster pastries and other baked goods. Less than 1 percent of the machines they looked at contained more nutritious foods like dried fruit, vegetables and yogurts, and exactly 0 percent of the machines contained fresh fruit or salads.[41] This is a problem, because people tend to buy whatever foods are on offer (duh), meaning that vending machines have the power to subconsciously shape people's nutritional habits.[42] If school vending machines only contain foods with poor nutritional value, then those are the foods that students will tend to eat.[43] On the flip side, if they were filled with more nutritious choices, it could positively benefit students' health. This is why governments sometimes intervene and mandate vending machines to contain healthier options, like the United States Department of Agriculture's "Smart Snacks in Schools" program, which limits foods containing excessive amounts of calories, sugars and fats.

Although these high-calorie snack dispensers are obviously common in schools,[44] they have also been considered as a possible point of concern in university campuses,[45] workplaces like healthcare facilities[46,47,48] and other public areas like train stations.[49] Basically, we humans tend to eat the foods that are most convenient to us, and having near-constant access to snacks is a modern obstacle that has had the power to radically transform our eating habits.

As an example of this, one research study tested if they could subconsciously shape consumers' eating habits in cafeterias by adopting the traffic light system used in some countries on food packaging to try to get them to buy more healthy "green" beverages like water, and fewer unhealthy "red" beverages like sugary soda.[50] On top of the color-coded traffic light system to encourage people to select the healthier drinks, they also rearranged the layout of the cafeteria so the preferable green drinks were more convenient, by placing them at eye level and also near the checkout, which was normally reserved for the sugary sodas. After six months, the cafeteria's soda sales decreased significantly in favor of water. If you can encourage people to eat more or less of certain foods just by changing how convenient they are to buy in one single cafeteria, imagine how profound the impact can be when you surround whole populations of people with high-calorie discretionary snacks in vending machines, gas stations, grocery store checkouts, cafes and food vendors.

## How Shops Can Subconsciously Influence Your Purchasing Patterns

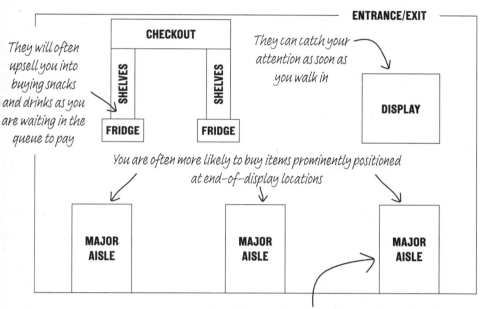

The items they want you to buy can also be positioned at eye-level throughout the store

### The rise of ultra-processed foods

Now that we are all in agreement that food has become more convenient, to the point where we are increasingly surrounded by it, we need to talk about the crux of this issue, which is food processing. If you walk into a large supermarket, you will see many foods that don't resemble anything that existed even 50 years ago. Cereals have evolved from a small number of basic and bland options to having a variety so massive that they now have their own aisle. Do you want a fruity-, caramel-, cinnamon- or chocolate-flavored breakfast? Don't worry, there are dozens to choose from. Some of them even contain marshmallows, cookie pieces or real chocolate fillings. Many of these "breakfast cereals" taste so good I am pretty sure they could be sold as desserts. There are also more aisles dedicated to snack foods like chips, candy, cookies, ice cream and soda. In addition, mega-profit-making food manufacturers employ teams of people to make these snacks irresistibly tasty, ensuring that, once you indulge, the taste compels you to keep coming back for more. They can manipulate how soft and creamy your ice cream tastes, how crunchy or gooey your cookies are, how sweet and flavorful your sodas are and how visually appealing your candy is, all in an attempt to increase their sales figures. If you feel like you can't stop eating these kinds of foods, that is because they are literally designed to produce this effect. Although the concept of "food addiction" is hotly debated, there is growing evidence that many ultra-processed foods are linked with addictive-like behaviors, such as having strong food cravings, consuming them in larger quantities than desired and struggling to cut down on eating them even if you want to do so.[51] If you think of foods that whisper in your subconscious to eat more of them, there is a strong possibility that the foods you think of are ultra-processed, like chocolate, cakes, doughnuts, ice cream and cookies.

It is important to understand that food processing isn't all "bad." In fact, processing has many benefits, including making products safer and more shelf-stable, so they can be cheaper for consumers.[52,53] For example, you can take naturally grown grains like corn and wheat and process them into cereals, breads and pastas, which are inexpensive, easily distributed and have long shelf lives, making them ideal for feeding vast populations. In times of food scarcity, this can literally save lives. Even ultra-processed foods are not always inherently *bad* as such—it is just an easy label to slap on a lot of industrially made, high-calorie and less nutritious food. For example, some research has shown that different subcategories are not actually linked with worse health, like ultra-processed wholegrain products not being associated with cardiometabolic risk factors like other ultra-processed foods,[54] or wholegrain and dairy products actually being linked with a reduced risk of type 2 diabetes,[55] or yogurt and dairy-based snacks being associated with a reduced risk of colorectal cancer in women.[56] However, as food processing has evolved, those same grains that gave us more nutritious foods like wholegrain breads and pastas, some of which are often still classed as "ultra-processed," have also given rise to a surge in tasty cookie shops, deep-fried doughnut franchises and vibrantly colored sugary soda conglomerates. Foods that are calorie-dense and hyperpalatable (a fancy term for "fucking delicious") now dominate our food supply. This change has inevitably caused collateral damage to our health, with diets high in ultra-processed foods being linked with a higher risk of adverse health outcomes, including dying earlier, dying earlier from heart disease specifically, obesity and cancer.[57] These high-calorie, nutrient-sparse ultra-processed foods have gradually started displacing more nutritious foods, and this dietary pattern shift looks like it is fucking up the health of our society. It's very hard to predict when this trend will stop because, metaphorically, once the toothpaste is out of the tube, it's very hard to push it back in. Trying to get people to eat fewer ultra-processed foods in favor of more fruits, vegetables, legumes (like beans, peas and lentils), lean proteins and wholegrains (like brown rice and oatmeal or wholemeal bread) is like trying to push a boulder up a hill, except that hill is getting steeper and more slippery as time goes on.

Although there is a surprising lack of research on how these foods impact our body weight, one research study tested what would happen if you gave people an entirely unprocessed diet or an entirely ultra-processed diet.[58] The participants lived in a facility where all the meals were precisely calculated and monitored to guarantee they would only eat the foods that were provided, but they were allowed to eat as much or as little of those foods as they wanted. When people were on the ultra-processed food diet they naturally consumed 508 calories more per day, which resulted in fat and weight gain. When people were on the unprocessed food diet, they naturally started losing body fat and weight, even though the study duration was only very short. Although "ultra-processed" is a huge umbrella term for a diverse group of foods, some of which are more nutritious, or more delicious, or more filling than others, the study shows that they tend to be worse for appetite regulation, on average. This shows us that eating more ultra-processed foods naturally encourages us to eat more energy, which nudges us toward gaining weight. Given these foods are becoming increasingly abundant in our food supply, it should not surprise anyone that society has been gradually gaining body fat. Funnily enough, in this study, the unprocessed diet cost nearly 50 percent more to create, which reinforces why many people are forced into eating lower quality diets based on what they can afford.

### Calorie Intake (top) and Body Weight Changes (bottom) During an Exclusively Ultra-Processed Diet and an Unprocessed Diet[59]

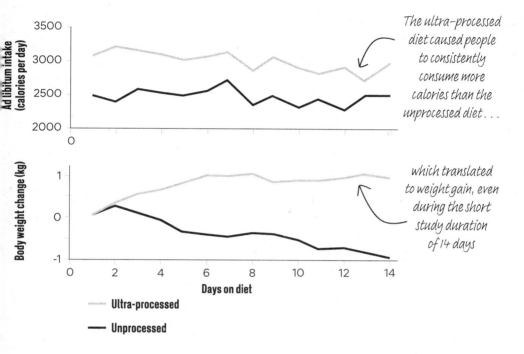

*The ultra-processed diet caused people to consistently consume more calories than the unprocessed diet . . .*

*which translated to weight gain, even during the short study duration of 14 days*

Ultra-processed
Unprocessed

### The role of advertising

When you step into your local supermarket, invariably you are immediately greeted by flashy signs and displays showcasing the newest food items on offer. They aren't the most nutritious options in the store, but many of them are actually cheaper than what you normally eat. Your mouth starts salivating because they look incredible, so you add a few to your basket. When you get home and try them, you discover that they are mind-blowingly tasty, and put your old favorite foods to shame. When you go back to the store, you are going to buy them again, right? This is one example of how food advertising can permeate your subconscious and subtly influence your food choices. Many other examples can be found in the media.

Can you think of a time where you were watching TV and you saw a food commercial with a close-up, slow-motion pour of an ice-cold soda, or someone cutting a pizza slice in overly dramatic lighting, or a juicy hamburger and fries that you know look a million times more aesthetic than if you actually bought them from your local fast-food drive-through? These are obvious forms of food advertising, but far more sneaky ones can be found in the form of product placement. You might be watching a film and see one of the main characters eating fast food with the logo showing or you are watching sports and your favorite athlete is sitting at a press conference where big soda companies pay to have their drinks conveniently sitting on their desk. Television food commercials have the power to immediately nudge children into consuming more food,[60] and this contributor to today's obesogenic environment has come under such scrutiny that the World Health Organization (WHO) has called for government restrictions on food and beverage marketing to children,[61] a bit like how the rules on cigarette and alcohol advertising directed at us adults are much stricter than they used to be. These are all little pieces of the puzzle that help explain why ultra-processed foods now make up the majority of the average person's diet, with some estimates putting this at nearly 60 percent for adults and 70 percent for adolescents.[62,63]

All of these factors are why the "obesity epidemic" should never be about pointing the finger of blame at you or any other individual, but instead viewed in the context of the wider changes that have driven our society toward gaining weight. For example, US government food subsidies can influence what foods are being produced and how much they cost.[64,65] This has led to an absolutely monumental shift in the overall US food market, which is now drowning in foods that can be manufactured to be tastier and more calorie-dense than ever. Although many factors can influence our body mass, this "push" of products into our food supply is thought by many to be the most powerful reason that we have been gaining weight as a society.[66,67] As we've discovered, these foods are also often cheaper than more nutritious options,[68,69] which makes it even more likely that you will pick them, especially if you don't have many pennies to spare in your bank account.

This is why, rather than blaming you for choosing the cheaper, tastier option, it's important for governments to focus on making healthier choices more affordable and more accessible in the first place.[70] This is like offering a $1 pack of gummy sweets and a $2 bag of spinach to a child and then blaming the child for not wanting to spend more of their pocket money to eat the far less tasty spinach. If anything, they are just succumbing to the innate human desire of wanting to eat something delicious, which also happens to be at a lower cost.

Basically, navigating our food environment is becoming an increasingly slippery landscape, but people still pin all the blame on you as the individual if you fall over. If maintaining good health is like swimming, the waters have been getting more treacherous over time and many of you feel like it's harder to stay afloat.

So, to revisit our earlier scenario, imagine you are a child born today compared to one hundred years ago. What factors are going to influence your propensity to gain weight? You aren't just choosing to eat more and exercise less because it sounds like a laugh. Instead, you exist in a totally different environment that has a much higher number of tasty, high-calorie, ultra-processed food options, more fast-food chains, more fast-food advertisements, larger portion sizes and more technology that encourages sedentary behavior. Although it is difficult to measure, it is of course possible that the dietary and exercise patterns you follow as a child will continue with you into adulthood.[71,72] For example, I was very physically active as a child and, as someone who loved playing sports, it was probably easier for me to feel comfortable joining a gym for the first time compared to someone who avoided all exercise classes in school because they were bullied about their weight, right?[73] Likewise, if you ate a lot of fast food as a child and never any fruits and vegetables, breaking those habits later in life is probably going to be trickier than for someone who has always eaten a nutritious diet.

## Childhood Obesity Causes

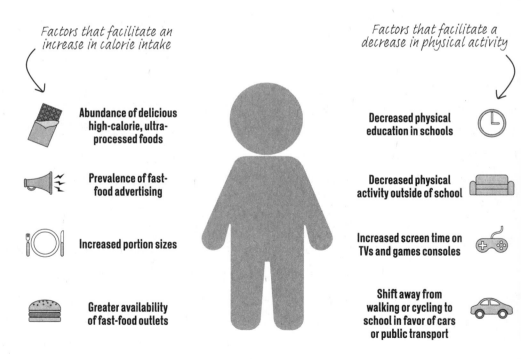

Factors that facilitate an increase in calorie intake

- Abundance of delicious high-calorie, ultra-processed foods
- Prevalence of fast-food advertising
- Increased portion sizes
- Greater availability of fast-food outlets

Factors that facilitate a decrease in physical activity

- Decreased physical education in schools
- Decreased physical activity outside of school
- Increased screen time on TVs and games consoles
- Shift away from walking or cycling to school in favor of cars or public transport

The point I really want to drive home is that you are always playing the cards you are dealt by the metaphorical casino dealer of life. From a health and body-weight perspective, the cards that most people are playing with today make it much more difficult to win the hand. This is not to say that it's impossible. It is just to reassure you that, if you are finding it difficult, please don't be too hard on yourself because you absolutely are not alone. Too many people spend their whole lives dieting, feeling shit when they struggle to stick to the diet plan and then blaming themselves for failing when they fall off the wagon. My goal for this book is to help you escape this cycle—by introducing fat loss habits that have been shown to work so you never have to buy a diet book again.

Before we explore those in Chapter 5, let's first discuss why so many of us find losing weight tricky in the first place.

# Why Losing Body Fat Is So F*cking Difficult

In theory, losing body fat is perfectly simple—you just eat less food and exercise more. Anyone who has restricted their food intake for even a brief period of time will probably say that they know how to diet. The difficult bit is actually keeping it off in the long run. As I have mentioned previously, anyone who goes on a diet inevitably loses weight temporarily, but a majority of people regain at least some of the weight they lost.[1,2]

## Weight loss versus fat loss

As a side note, although I talk about "weight loss," most people actually care about losing body fat, specifically. You can technically lose weight by sitting in a sauna and taking a bunch of laxatives, but the weight you lose will just be water through sweating and the contents of your gastrointestinal tract through diarrhea, which aren't things you should feel excited about losing. Although weight loss and fat loss aren't always the same thing, people who lose a lot of body fat tend to weigh less than they did previously. Also, because it is easy to measure how much you weigh by standing on the scale but it is difficult to precisely measure how much body fat you have, "weight loss" is actually the more popular term. Consider losing weight and losing body fat as closely related siblings, but losing weight unfortunately gets far more attention than losing body fat.

Knowing that diets often have a shitty success rate in the long term should not really be counterintuitive. After all, if weight regain *wasn't* common then people could just go on a single diet, lose body fat once and then live happily ever after at their new post-diet weight, right? But we all instinctively know that the likelihood of this is only a touch above me suddenly being elected the next US president.

If you have ever struggled to lose weight, I can bet good money that someone somewhere has made you feel like you should find it easier than you do. People who are naturally thin may tell you that you just need to "eat less food and do more exercise" as if this is anything more helpful than stating the profoundly obvious. If you were a football (or soccer, for American readers) player and you were on a painfully long losing streak, imagine someone coming over to you and telling you that winning is easy if you just "concede fewer goals and score more." Alternatively, imagine you have been really struggling to support your family financially and someone tells you that you just need to "spend less and save more." While all of this advice is technically correct, it is so painfully obvious that it is about as useful as a snowplow in the Sahara Desert.

Someone who doesn't understand your position probably isn't

the best person to give you empathetic advice. So, let's do something that most weight loss books never ever do and roll back the curtain on *why* losing weight (and maintaining the loss) can actually be really fucking difficult.

## The Genetics of Fat Storage

Some people think that genetics does not play a role in how much body fat you store. I have seen countless social media videos featuring personal trainers saying things like, "It's not your genetics' fault that you are fat!," and those videos invariably want me to bang my head against a wall with increasing intensity because they don't give the full picture. If I had to pick just one word for people who make claims like this, it would probably be something like frustratinglyignorantplusalsoquiteannoying.

Genetics can be a super complex topic, so I am just going to give you an express summary and hope I can teach you a little bit without making you so bored you decide to close this book.

The link between genetics and weight is by no means a new discovery. Even research papers from one hundred years ago noted that children tend to inherit similar physiques to their parents, finding that slenderness, for example, often "runs in families."[3] Now, it is entirely possible that children often look like their parents because they have similar lifestyles, right? For example, if both parents are avid "junk food"-avoiding, green-juice-smoothie-drinking, let's-all-go-hiking-before-breakfast kind of people, we would probably guess that their children would grow up to be more active and perhaps thinner than the average human. That being said, if breeds of animals can vary by shape and size because of genetics, surely the same applies to people?

Dating right back to the 1950s, research papers have tried to answer this question by looking at sets of twins, allowing them to estimate just how much genetics plays a role in how much body fat you have.[4,5] For example, if you look at sets of identical and non-identical twins over a 25-year period, you will notice that their body shapes are strongly influenced by genetics,[6] even when those twins are raised apart rather than growing up in the same household.[7] This is in line with other research papers, which concluded that children who had been adopted often had similar body weights to their biological parents rather than their adoptive parents.[8,9]

Basically, how you eat and how you exercise can obviously change how much you weigh, but how much body fat you have and where you store it is often at least vaguely similar to that of your parents, even if they did not raise you in the same way they were raised. Did you ever know someone who was naturally intelligent even if they didn't try hard at school, or naturally good at sports they hadn't even tried before? Well, similarly, some people are probably genetically predisposed to being naturally thinner than others.

How does this relate to body fat? Think of it like this: if you were naturally very short as a child, it's going to be harder for you to become the next basketball star than for the rare subset of people who are approaching 2m (6½ft) tall. Sometimes genetics can be difficult or even impossible to change. Likewise, there are rare genetic conditions, which often develop in early childhood, where young kids are predisposed to gaining a significant amount of weight extremely quickly.[10] Most commonly, though, genetics are more like dimmer switches where you might be subtly better or worse at things without it being as obvious—for example, you could be a similar height, but you've never been able to throw a basketball with as much ease as the genetically gifted child prodigy. The most common genetic influences of obesity are harder for other people to see—like having significantly higher appetite levels driving you toward eating more food—but they still make a big difference to how much body fat you store and how easy you find dieting.[11]

As an example of this, my wife and I own two dogs. One of them is a chihuahua and one is a pug. As many dog owners will attest, pugs are renowned for being constantly hungry. It doesn't matter if you have just fed our pug, he will still act as if he is starving. Every time you are cooking, he will be there by your feet hopefully waiting for you to accidentally drop something. Every time you are eating, he will be there staring at you, hoping you might give him a mouthful. It doesn't matter if he is sound asleep in your lap, if he hears someone open a packet of food, he will leap off you and forget you exist. I would bet good money that, if you left him alone in a food pantry, he would eat himself to death, and probably do it with no regrets. On the other hand, our chihuahua is often very ambivalent about food. You can give her breakfast and, on some days, she will sniff it and walk away. Genetically, our pug is always hungry and, yes, we can make him lose or gain weight depending on how much food we give him, but if he was in charge of his own food, he would happily eat himself into an early grave. This is an animal example of the term "food noise," where some humans report "heightened and/or persistent manifestations of food cue reactivity, often leading to food-related intrusive thoughts and maladaptive eating behaviors."[12] Some of you might notice that you are in a near-perpetual state of hunger, something you might feel like you are fighting constantly that makes you far more susceptible to overeating, but this is invisible to other people. They might just think you are lazy, or view you as gluttonous, rather than realizing there are biological reasons your appetite is higher than theirs.

People often dismiss the role of genetics because obesity is more common nowadays. If genetics *causes* people to have more body fat, why wasn't this affecting populations one hundred years ago? Well, imagine you have a genetically higher appetite than I do, for example. If you constantly feel hungrier than me, and need to eat a lot more food before you start feeling full, are you more susceptible to gaining weight than I am? Of course you are. This genetic difference becomes more obvious when the foods on offer change. As we discussed in the last chapter, overeating was significantly harder one hundred years ago when mouthgasmic calorie-dense foods were rarer than rocking horse shit—unlike today's food environment. This is why experts often say, "Genetics loads the gun, but the environment pulls the trigger."[3]

Basically, while genetics is a hugely complicated subject, it shouldn't be controversial to acknowledge that some people find it considerably harder to lose body fat than others. I have worked with people who can reduce their calorie intake as easily as taking a gentle walk in the park. I have also worked with others who feel like their appetite levels are so naturally high that trying to reduce what they eat feels more like running uphill, except the hill is actually a mountain, and the mountain is on fire.

## What Happens When You Lose Body Fat

For a moment, let's pretend that you have just eaten the biggest lunch of your life. You have been to an all-you-can-eat buffet and absolutely chowed down, eating anything and everything in sight. You feel so stuffed that the idea of even one more mouthful of food is enough to make you feel a little bit nauseous. In a few hours when dinnertime rolls around, it's quite likely that you don't want to eat your normal portion, right?

Now let's reverse that. Imagine you woke up late for work this morning and you didn't have time to eat your usual breakfast before you rushed out the door. When lunchtime arrives, you pull out your normal lunch you brought from home and realize it has gone moldy, so you have nothing to eat. You have accidentally skipped two meals, so, when dinnertime finally arrives, you feel absolutely ravenous, and you are ready to chew your own arm off. Do you eat your usual portion? No, your hunger has increased to compensate for your missed meals, and you eat a much bigger dinner than usual.

This is a very short-term example of how your body can naturally adjust how hungry it is based on how much food you have eaten; a process that is outside of your conscious control. Now, it's possible that this concept can be extended into the long term as well. For example, if you diet for a few weeks, your hunger levels can creep up and naturally encourage your body to start eating more food again.

Strangely, one of the best ways of testing this concept is in rodents—you can precisely measure their food and give them more or less for a period of time to see what happens, whereas keeping humans locked in cages to do the same thing poses a bit more of an ethical dilemma to researchers. After a series of experiments in the 1940s, researchers noticed that rats adapted their natural food intake depending on whether they had been under- or overfed.[14] Essentially, they discovered that, if they tinkered around with an area of the rat's brain called the hypothalamus, they could stimulate its appetite so much that it would suddenly want to keep eating food and gain more body fat. However, when they put that rat on a bland diet to reduce its calorie intake, the rat would lose weight, but this would also induce "voracious" hunger and the rat would start eating more food until it went back to its original size. Have you ever dieted and lost weight but suddenly felt so fucking hungry all the time that it became impossible to stick to the diet you were currently on? Well, that.

## What Is "Set Point" Theory? A Simplified Explanation

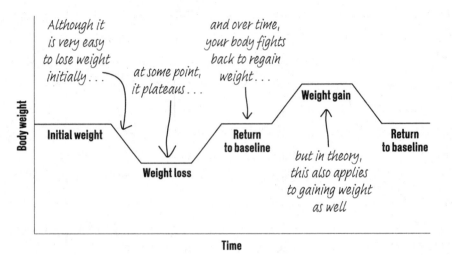

This research on rats is where the phenomenon known as the "set point" theory began, the idea that you will probably lose and gain weight periodically throughout your life, but that your body has inbuilt mechanisms that always return you to your normal, or "set point," weight.[15]

Having a precise "set point" does not make sense in the real world, though. If you eat a lot more food over the holiday period and gain weight, will your appetite suddenly drop to the point you return to your exact starting weight? No. If your body *always* returned to its exact starting weight, nobody would continue to gain weight throughout their lifetime, but we know that this obviously isn't the case.[16] It would also make long-term weight loss literally impossible, but we know that many people are able to lose weight and successfully keep it off in the long term, even if it's not the majority of people.[17]

Although the set point theory is flawed, it is still true that your body has certain adaptation mechanisms in place that can make losing weight a progressively trickier mountain to climb, even if it's hard to pinpoint exactly what these are.[18,19] What we know for sure is that, when people lose weight, it's very common for their appetite to increase, which can obviously make sticking to a reduced-calorie diet progressively harder.[20,21] After all, existing on less food when your hunger is higher than it used to be sounds like an express train straight to the land of misery and despair, doesn't it? We also know that, as people lose weight, their body also tends to burn less energy.[22,23] If you have a large dog and a small dog, the small dog will invariably require less food than the big dog, unless the small dog is training for a doggy-marathon, of course. Likewise, a very small car tends to require much less fuel to make a journey than a huge truck, right? Generally speaking, smaller things require less energy to exist and to move than their larger counterparts. If you want to continue gaining weight for the rest of your life, you can't just eat 5 percent more than you do now forevermore—you would need to continually eat more food to facilitate continual weight gain. Therefore, if your goal is to lose body fat and lose weight from where you are now, you are going to incrementally require fewer calories to maintain your body weight than you do now. So, if you have ever been on a diet, lost weight rapidly at first and then found it harder and harder to keep it off, you are not a failure. You are among a huge group of people who have realized just how difficult dieting can be.

If you are not convinced by this physiological phenomenon, please keep in mind that even after people lose a lot of weight by using strong medications that help suppress appetite, or even following bariatric surgery procedures, there are people who still regain a significant amount of the weight they originally lost.[24,25,26] It's important to remember that this is an average—there are some people who do significantly better and some who do significantly worse. This is not to say that long-term weight loss is impossible, which is a harmful narrative to reinforce. It is simply explaining why some people struggle so much. This is why developing healthy long-term habits that become second nature can help you combat this negative yo-yo dieting cycle.

## Body Weight Change in Response to Semaglutide Injections (2.4mg per week) and Subsequent Follow-up Period[27]

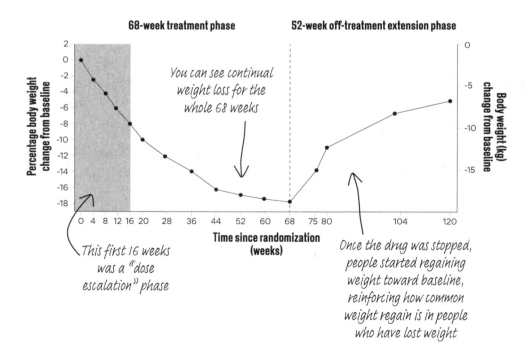

## Your Weight Is Not a Behavior

I like to think of your weight and how much body fat you store as something you are not fully in control of but, instead, something you can influence to varying degrees. They are more like a by-product of a shitload of factors, some of which you can change and some of which you can't.

As a metaphor, let's swap your weight for another physical trait, like your skin. As a teenager, I suffered with some pretty bad acne. I tried all kinds of different creams, gels, patches and exfoliating scrubs to try to get clearer skin, including some potent stuff my doctor prescribed me. At best, they were like squirting a water pistol onto a burning building. I was so self-conscious that I would often walk around trying not to make eye contact with anyone. As I grew up and my teenage hormonal fluctuations calmed the fuck down, the frequency of angry-looking spots on my face subsided, despite the fact that I was spending less on skincare than I did previously.

Fast-forward to my mid-30s: I was having a chat with my wife and one of our best friends, when our friend asked my wife what skincare products she used to achieve such an incredibly smooth complexion. My wife laughed and said, "I wash my face with water, and that's about it." She always had effortlessly great skin without having to invest in any of the various potions that either my friend or I had tried. See, you can obviously do things to improve how your skin looks, but ultimately you are still playing the cards that the genetic lottery has dealt you, right?

So, what influences how much body fat you store? Obviously, your genetics and individual biology can play a big part. What foods you eat and how much exercise you do can also play a major role, but many lesser-known factors also have the ability to subconsciously influence this. For example, environmental and economic factors can make a difference, like what foods are available to you where you live and what you can afford. If your personal financial situation looks bleaker than the winter weather forecast in England, you are unlikely to be spending a lot of money on expensive organic green smoothies. If you live in the rural countryside surrounded by thriving farmland, you might find it easier to eat fresh, locally grown produce, or if you live by the coast, you might find it easier to eat affordable fish and seafood than someone who lives in the arsehole of nowhere in the middle of a big country can. Although it's difficult to precisely quantify, if your environment determines the kinds of foods you can afford to buy, this could have a secondary effect on your health and body weight.[28,29] In the same way that growing up in a busy city with a lot of pollution can impact your lung health, your surroundings can also shape what you eat and how active you are, sometimes without you even realizing it.

Psychological factors can also make a difference. For example, if you are someone who constantly "comfort eats" in response to life stress, this obviously has the power to promote weight gain, right? After all, we humans often tend to reach for high-sugar and high-fat foods when we feel emotional, which is why some research papers have examined the effectiveness of adopting alternative coping mechanisms to help decrease the risk of continual weight gain,[30] which we will talk about in more detail in Chapter 6. This is an example of why people with depression or severe mental illness often have a higher risk of obesity.[31,32]

At its core, the reason some people mistakenly think that losing or gaining weight is easy-peasy is because it hinges on two simple things that sound like they are fully within your control: what you eat and how much you exercise. However, actual authorities on the topic are far more aware of all those sneaky subliminal factors that influence these. For example, the WHO has an "acceleration plan to stop obesity," which doesn't just say, "Tell more people to diet and exercise, and everything will be fine," but instead acknowledges the complex genetic, environmental and psychosocial factors that can influence your nutrition and exercise behaviors.[33] The people who know the most about the topic are the first to admit that this shit is complicated, and that losing weight is not always super straightforward for various reasons.

As losing weight is not a super-easy end result that you can simply snap your fingers to effortlessly achieve, I think it is a good idea to reframe what you should be paying most attention to.

## Focus On the Behaviors Rather Than Obsessing Over the Outcomes

Imagine you are a dentist and one hundred of your patients all told you that they wanted to have a perfect Hollywood-esque smile. We're talking teeth so blindingly white that you need sunglasses to be in the same room as them. You would already know that, for some of them, this is a tad unrealistic, and probably not a goal most people could achieve without paying a lot of money to get some fancy teeth veneers. If all of your patients obsess over the outcome of wanting their teeth to look perfect, some of them will inevitably be disappointed if they can't get there. However, you also know that it is entirely possible for all of them to improve their dental health without needing to resort to drastic measures.

If my original outcome goal is to improve my dental health, what would you tell me? You would probably break this down into key individual behaviors and habits. For example, there are habits you would want me to do more of, like making sure I am brushing and flossing regularly. There are some habits you might want me to do less of, like consuming foods that stain my teeth directly before bed or grinding my teeth when I sleep. There are also some behaviors you would want me to ideally stop doing completely, like the terrible party trick I have of opening beer bottles using only my teeth, because that's clearly not a smart idea, and I have the teeth chips to prove it.

When it comes to losing weight, or losing body fat specifically, it is extraordinarily common for people to pluck unrealistic goals out of the air and then feel like dog shit if they can't hit them.[34,35] Obsessing over the outcome goal is also not a smart idea because it fails to take into consideration how you will get there and also how you will feel in the process. Let's say your friend has a goal to lose 4.5kg (10lb) in a month. If they manage to lose that amount of weight, are they happy? On paper, yes. But what if they reached that weight by resorting to a horribly restrictive crash diet? What if they followed a diet they hated, cut out all of their favorite foods, swapped their main meals for weight loss shakes, choked down some green smoothies that tasted like grass mixed with sadness and bought some dodgy weight loss pills from the shady-looking guy in the gym? They may have hit their goal weight, but if they can't sustain it and they feel dreadful in the process, is it really a win? I propose not.

Too many people focus on getting to the destination without pausing to consider how they feel on the journey. This is a very common issue when it comes to dieting specifically, where people often engage in unhealthy weight loss strategies. These can range from mild to far more severe, such as skipping meals, consuming excessive amounts of caffeine for appetite suppression, taking diet pills or laxatives, or even vomiting.[36] People who engage in these kinds of extreme behaviors are often more likely to be susceptible to weight regain,[37] eating disorders[38] and depression,[39] even to the point it can be severe to life-threatening.[40] We will talk about goal-setting in a lot more detail in Chapter 4 to help you steer clear of these kinds of pitfalls.

The key takeaway is: rather than being so obsessed about getting from A to B that you feel you need to resort to extreme, potentially harmful tactics to help you get there, it makes sense to focus on healthy behaviors that make your journey feel as pleasant as possible. If you hit a weight loss goal but your physical and mental health have been drop-kicked off a building in the process, it's not the victory you originally hoped for.

Before we move on to dietary strategies and individual habits in the following chapters, let's start shifting our attention on to you so we can begin creating a plan of attack that is actually customized for your own circumstances and preferences.

## Identifying Your Barriers and Facilitators

If you wanted help with something you were seriously struggling with and you sat down to talk with a therapist, they definitely would not start off your very first session by telling you what you should do to feel happier and improve your quality of life, because at that point they know absolutely fuck all about you. Instead, they would ask you questions, let you talk and try to get to the bottom of whatever it is that is bothering you in the first place.

So, let's do the same thing, and break this down into more practical examples so you can identify any obstacles you need to overcome.

Although many people go on a diet and are unsuccessful in the long term, there are actually studies with much better success rates, where around half of participants were still maintaining a clinically significant degree of weight loss five to eight years after the initial weight loss phase.[41,42] This is in stark contrast with some very bleak-looking research papers where only 5 percent of dieters were classed as "successful" in the long term.[43] The research studies with better success rates are inevitably a lot more hands-on and are often described as "interdisciplinary" or "multidisciplinary" and don't just include diet plans, but often structured and progressive exercise programs, psychological help like behavioral therapy (we will discuss some psychological concepts in Chapter 6), plus follow-up appointments with relevant professionals. Ongoing support is key. Imagine I trained you and your identical twin. If you were both given the exact same exercise program, but your twin was just handed it on a piece of paper whereas I saw you once a week or once a month to keep you accountable and assess your progress, I would bet good money that you would get much better long-term results than they would.

One of the biggest lessons we can learn from these examples is that handing people a diet plan and metaphorically kicking them out the door is terrible practice. When this is how weight loss programs are prescribed, their success rates tend to be atrocious. If you have ever been handed a diet plan or told what you should eat and then been waved on your way with no further support, the statistical likelihood of you sticking with the plan for decades is nearly non-existent. On the other hand, more comprehensive advice can be very useful. So, imagine you are hiring me as your personal trainer but instead of me telling you to eat less food and exercise more, I actually sit down with you and ask you what you are struggling with and why. If we can identify your obstacles, maybe we can find a way to overcome them together.

For example, what are the actual reasons someone finds themselves eating more food or struggling to get to the gym? Studies exploring these causes have uncovered potential barriers, such as food-related emotional regulation—for example, people who ate more food not because they were hungry, but because they self-soothed certain emotions, like anxiety, loneliness or depression. People who regained weight after a diet phase often reported binge eating triggered by negative thoughts, rather than hunger.[44] Researchers have actually used an algorithm solely for people who were struggling to keep up with their gym routine.[45] So, if you said, "Hey Ben, I have been struggling to keep up with my workouts recently," it wouldn't be helpful for me to say, "Just do them, you lazy piece of shit," but it would be helpful to find a strategy that helps you overcome any barriers you are facing.

Do you dislike exercising on your own? In which case, would you enjoy exercising with a friend? Would you feel more motivated in a group setting, like joining an exercise class where you might also make friends who can make your workouts more enjoyable? Are you unsure of what to do? In which case, would you benefit from having a workout plan given to you, like a video you can play where someone demonstrates what exercises you can follow? Do you feel like you need to see a personal trainer regularly to help with your accountability and make you feel more comfortable in the gym? Would you prefer exercising at home? In which case, do you need some equipment to use to help you have effective workouts? Do you hate walking, jogging or running because they are uncomfortable? In which case, would better fitting clothing or more appropriate footwear help? These are examples of actual problem-solving questions and strategies to try to help when someone is simply not finding it easy to exercise regularly. If I can help make exercise more enjoyable and decrease any unnecessary discomfort, you have a much better shot at keeping that exercise routine going, right? Not everyone naturally loves working out, but there are things you can tweak and change to at least make it less unpleasant than walking barefoot across hot coals.

Let's extend this thought process outside of exercising and steer it toward overall diet, lifestyle and weight loss changes. There are research papers that ask people to identify their own barriers and facilitators that make losing weight more or less difficult.[46,47,48] In Chapters 4–6, we will drill down to help you create an action plan based on your own unique preferences and circumstances. For the moment, the following is a very abridged list of barriers and facilitators that can impact your diet, physical activity levels or weight loss in general.

Obviously, as you are reading this book, I am not in the same room with you (if I am, one of us should probably call the police), so I cannot work with you specifically, but I can list out the most common roadblocks and motivators and you can mentally check them in your head to see if some of them might apply to you.

These can be broken down into separate groups, so let's use three simple ones:

1. Individual internal factors. For example, do you feel motivated as you read this book?
2. Social and environmental factors. For example, do you have friends that influence your food choices?

3. Program-specific factors. For example, someone gives you a workout and diet plan that you could love, or you could hate.

### Individual internal factors

Of course, it makes sense that if you really fucking want something, you are more likely to chase it. I will happily get in my car and drive ten minutes to a shop for cookies if they are delicious enough, but I am reluctant to walk ten steps into my kitchen to get the lettuce out of the fridge, wash it and chop it up to make a salad. The most common factors that influence someone's initial motivation to change their lifestyle include improving pre-existing health conditions, decreasing the likelihood of health conditions they are at a high risk of, wanting to live longer, participating in important relationships and setting good examples for loved ones. Some motivational factors may also change with age. For example, teenagers may be more inclined to start working out for aesthetic reasons or to avoid weight-related bullying,[49] but as people get older, they are often more inclined to exercise to promote well-being and slow down aging, like staying strong and mobile so they can go on holidays and take care of loved ones later in life.[50] Deep-rooted motivations often have a lot longer on their expiration date than fleeting aesthetic goals. If you have children and you desperately want to be in good health so you can live long enough to play with your grandkids, you will probably willingly use your gym membership much more consistently over a longer period of time than someone who joins the gym simply because they want to lose weight for their wedding that is 12 weeks away.

Once you start exercising, seeing your body change is often reported as a very positive motivational tool, which sounds great, but it also means the reverse is true. If you stop seeing your body changing as quickly, then your motivation levels can suddenly drop faster than a sack of potatoes being thrown off a building. Unfortunately, many people only exercise for weight loss purposes, so they judge its usefulness exclusively by whether they see the number on the scales going down. This is a problem because, even if you do lose weight, you cannot lose weight forever. You would literally die, which would be a major buzzkill. Despite that, one of the most common reasons to abandon exercise like an unwanted birthday gift is because the number on the scales stops moving.[51] If you *only* judge how effective a workout plan is by whether or not you lose weight, you may accidentally overlook a whole host of physical and mental health benefits that may be invisible to the naked eye. This is why having other goals that excite you is a smart idea. Seeing yourself getting stronger, feeling yourself getting fitter, noticing your quality of life improving or noticing your mental health getting better are all encouraging pats on the back that make you feel good and nudge you to want to keep going long after the quick goal like "lose a few pounds by this summer" expires. So, do yourself a favor and think about having other, meaningful long-term goals.

### Social and environmental factors

One of the most commonly reported factors for whether someone finds it easier to lose weight in the long term is social support.[52] If you have supportive friends and family, this can make it much easier to continue. Going to the gym can be a lot more fun if your best friend loves going with you. Eating healthily is a lot easier if you live with a partner who also enjoys the same food as you. The flip side is also true; if the people closest to you are saboteurs, and make you feel guilty for wanting to exercise or eat healthily, it can make it harder for you, especially if you are a friendly, people-pleasing kind of person. Even little things like whether you own a dog or not can make a significant difference in how willing you are to go for a walk.[53] The likelihood of me leaving my house on my own just to go for a casual stroll is half a smidge above zero, but going for a walk with my wife and our dogs is very pleasant and I happily do it daily. Unsurprisingly, the weather and what nature is easily available are also reported barriers and facilitators for how active people are.[54] Since moving to Southern California, I can see more people exercising outside in a single day than I would where I used to live in England for a whole month. After all, playing volleyball on the beach in the sun is fun, but jogging outside when it's cold, gloomy and pissing down with rain is about as appealing as going for a swim in shark-infested waters. This is especially true if you live in an unsafe area because nobody really wants to go out for an inner-city jog if they think there is a decent chance they will get robbed, right?

Other big environmental factors can be things like what food you can afford in your local area, how easy it is for you to get to your nearest gym and what food surrounds you on a daily basis. If you work sitting down at a desk for 12 hours a day surrounded by high-calorie, delicious treats, or your work cafeteria provides your food, these factors clearly have the power to shape your daily activity levels and food choices. I don't eat many cakes and pastries, but if I worked in a bakery, I guarantee that would change faster than you can say "double chocolate cheesecake."

Social and environmental factors are always going to be present and sometimes they are difficult to overcome, but being aware of them can be useful. For example, you can make changes to your immediate food environment to make it more conducive to your goals, which we will discuss in Chapter 5 when we look at the healthy habits for long-term fat loss.

## Program-specific factors

Obviously, if someone writes you a workout program or diet plan that you detest, you probably aren't going to willingly do it for the rest of your life. So, to kick things off, let's throw shitty, overly restrictive diet plans and workout programs straight in the bin. Also, if I write you a training program that requires you to go to the gym three times per week, but you don't have any gyms that are conveniently located near you (or if you hate those gyms because they are full of arseholes), that is a possible barrier to completing the program versus me writing you a program you could complete at home. On the flip side, if you are a member of a sports or dance class that you love going to because it's convenient, and you are friends with other members who go there, these are facilitators that make you much more likely to stick with the program. This is how the program you follow can also amplify the very important social support aspect we have already talked about. Having support from knowledgeable professionals (like personal trainers and dietitians) can understandably be useful for accountability,[55] and having an ongoing way of checking in and monitoring your progress can be helpful too—like using food diaries[56] or tracking your step count with a pedometer,[57] both of which we will be discussing in more detail shortly. Many people struggle with the feeling of being "cast away" without any ongoing support, which is part of the reason why weight loss groups are so popular, rather than someone just handing you a diet plan and wishing you the best of luck.

Some of the above barriers are not things you can change, or are things you cannot change very easily (if you can control the weather or how much fruit and vegetables cost, you are obviously blessed with a higher power), but some of them are things that you will be able to find solutions to or workarounds for. So do yourself a favor and focus on the things that are within your capabilities.

For example, a few years ago, one of my best friends told me he struggled to have the same "discipline" to go to the gym as I did. If he trained three times per week and I trained six times per week, it made sense to think that I was more dedicated, on the surface. But that is the risk of judging things at face value. My friend was a father of two children. He used to wake up before 6am to start his long commute to work, where he tended to work overtime hours, and then have another painful drive home in rush-hour traffic. When he got home he made sure to spend the majority of his time with his wife and kids, so he told me the only time he would go to the gym was after 9pm, because that's around when both of his children would fall asleep. He told me that having the willpower to go to the gym after he had been reading his kids a bedtime story in a dark room was extremely hard because, of course, his body was also desperately wanting to wind down for bedtime. Me? I was a self-employed personal trainer. I had no children to take care of so I could exercise whatever time of the day I wanted. I used to literally book my clients around my preferred hours just to make sure I had time to train and, as I worked in a gym, squeezing exercise into my daily routine was about as easy as easy can be. He viewed me as having more discipline when, in reality, he had far bigger obstacles than I did and I had far more facilitators stacking in my favor than he did. He didn't lack discipline at all.

If anything, his day-to-day life was far harder than mine, and that is precisely why it was easier for me to work out.

Some of his barriers toward a healthier and happier life were very difficult to overcome, like finding a job that paid as well as his current job but was more local to him. But from an exercise perspective, his main barriers were lack of time and energy because he was a busy father working hard to provide and care for his family, so he was permanently fucking exhausted. Training in the evenings wasn't a sustainable long-term solution, so he managed to find a convenient and affordable gym he could train at on his lunch hour when he had more energy, and I helped write a short program he could squeeze into a very brief time period. He worked with the circumstances he had to find the best solution.

Why is this section so important? Very simply, because if there are possible obstacles in your life that make things harder, understanding what they are gives you a far better chance of adopting and maintaining healthy habits. There are a shitload of research papers solely dedicated to the reasons people find sticking with diets and workout programs hard, so let's agree that, if you are struggling to follow something consistently, this does not mean you are broken. It means you are human, with complex circumstances, and the best way to make an appropriate, personalized plan for you is to understand those circumstances and work with them rather than feeling like a failure because you might be finding things difficult.

In the following chapters, we will discuss different dietary approaches so you can find something that works for you, as well as giving you a menu of healthy habits you can handpick to suit your own individual circumstances, allowing you to build a customized strategy that gives you the best chance of long-term success.

## Commonly Reported Barriers and Facilitators to Diet, Exercise and Weight Loss

| Barriers | Example(s) |
|---|---|
| Lack of initial motivation | If you have struggled with yo-yo dieting throughout your life, making nutrition changes or rejoining a gym can feel daunting. If you have a lot going on, exercise often takes a back seat to other priorities. |
| Lack of time and energy | Trying to squeeze exercise into long work hours or a hectic family life when you already feel exhausted can be extremely difficult. |
| Lack of enjoyment | Being given a terrible crash diet and exercise plan you detest that rapidly removes your will to live doesn't exactly make you want to keep going. |
| Lack of money | Unable to afford local gym memberships or at-home equipment. Struggling to afford nutritious foods when less nutritious foods are often cheaper. |
| Lack of support | Being given a program and then kicked out the door without any ongoing guidance or accountability. |
| Lack of personalization | Being given a copy-and-paste training regimen and meal plan that don't suit your personal preferences. |
| Lack of results | If you cannot see physical changes from working out, it can be significantly less exciting to keep going unless you can find another reward that makes you want to continue. |
| Sickness | Physical disability can make exercising anything from more difficult to impossible, especially if you are in a lot of pain. |
| Saboteurs | Partners, family or friends that proactively discourage you from doing what you want or make you feel guilty. |
| Weight stigma | Receiving negative comments about your weight. Being injured or mocked in the gym, which makes you less likely to want to keep going. |
| Inner food cues | Eating for reasons besides hunger, like eating a lot when bored, stressed, anxious or sad. |
| Dichotomous thinking | An all-or-nothing mindset that makes you want to give up the moment you deviate slightly from a plan, like eating one cookie and then thinking "Fuck it, my whole diet is ruined." |

| Facilitators | Example(s) |
|---|---|
| **High initial motivation** | Exercising frequently is much easier when you enjoy doing it, or have a deep-rooted motivation like wanting to improve your health, lower disease risk or extend your healthy years on this planet so you can spend more time with loved ones. |
| **Ongoing motivation** | Noticing physical changes often feels motivating, but they are often also very slow to see. It is very rare to see noticeable changes weekly, so having other ongoing sources of motivation can be great, like feeling yourself getting fitter, healthier or stronger. |
| **Social support** | Exercising regularly can be a lot easier if you have people who also like to exercise with you, like friends, family or even strangers when it is in a group class setting because socializing can be nice. Access to professionals like a personal trainer can also be helpful. |
| **Psychological improvement** | Ongoing sources of motivation don't have to be physical. A lot of people who turn exercising into an ingrained habit do so because of psychological changes, like having better mental health, feeling more confident or noticing improved mood. |
| **Having a clear, personalized plan** | Actually knowing what you are doing can make it easier to move forward. For example, a plan devised specifically for you by a personal trainer versus walking around the gym aimlessly, or some clear nutrition habits that suit your personal preferences. |
| **Conducive exercise environment** | Being physically active can be much easier when you live or work in an area that facilitates it, like having a gym next to your workplace or having safe walking routes by your home. |
| **Conducive food environment** | Making dietary changes can be easier when preferred foods are more accessible, like having affordable nutritious foods offered by your workplace and convenience stores close to your home. |
| **Psychological flexibility** | Instead of all-or-nothing thinking where you feel like your plan is ruined every time you deviate from it even slightly, knowing that you can keep progressing forward is important. You don't need to be perfect to keep showing up and making progress. |
| **Self-monitoring** | People who monitor their progress and behaviors often see better long-term results, like people who are successful in business may be more inclined to frequently check their bank balance. This may include weighing yourself regularly or keeping a nutrition and training diary. |

# 3

# Exploring Different Diet Types

Weight loss diets tend to generate cult-like followings. Regardless of which one you pick, you will find whole books and social media groups dedicated to promoting that specific diet, and die-hard followers who believe that their method is the absolute best way of eating for everyone. So, first things first, we need to set the record straight.

There is no "best" diet for everyone. Think of it like choosing a car; if you walk into a Ford garage, the salesperson will happily tell you all the reasons you should buy a Ford, but if you walk into the Audi garage down the road, you will immediately be told that an Audi is in fact the best car for you. The honest truth is, there is no universally perfect car. If I were one of those dogmatic petrolheads who went out of their way to persuade you that their car was the best on the planet, you would rightfully view me as being an irritating little shitbag. Yet, that is how most people talk about diets. And even if you *did* like the same car as me, that doesn't mean you have to love everything about it, right? You can love an exotic sports car for how it looks and how fast it goes, but still acknowledge that driving long journeys in it is less comfortable than someone dragging you down a cobbled street by your ankles. In order to make the smartest decisions for yourself, you need to assess the pros and cons—and diets are no exception.

To help drive this point home (pardon the car pun), in 2014 a review paper published in the *Journal of the American Medical Association* (*JAMA*) noted that many diets advertise themselves to you as being superior, but we don't actually know which of them is genuinely best, so they pooled lots of research studies together to see which could be crowned as the champion.[1] They included 48 different controlled trials with over 7,000 participants to finally answer which diet reigns supreme. The results were very anticlimactic. Despite including a wide array of different branded diets like Atkins, Zone, Ornish, Slimming World, Weight Watchers, South Beach, Rosemary Conley, Jenny Craig and Volumetrics, none of them could be seen as victorious. The differences in success between each of them were so small that the researchers claimed that the diet you follow was of "little importance," and this supports the idea that the specific diet doesn't matter much, and you should just pick something you can actually stick to.

These kinds of research studies will often put two diets head-to-head to see which one wins. For example, if group A go on a low-carb diet and group B go on a low-fat diet, who loses the most weight after 12 weeks? While this sounds great in theory, it has taken decades to reach the surprisingly underwhelming conclusion that it probably doesn't matter that fucking much (which is me paraphrasing, obviously). If you took all those individual weight loss studies and lined them up to find a clear winner, no diet would stand head and shoulders above the rest. This doesn't just apply to branded diets like Slimming World, Atkins, Zone and Weight Watchers, which have different macronutrient ratios (some are lower in fat, some are lower in carbohydrates),[2,3] it also includes non-branded meal-timing diets, like intermittent fasting,[4] and can even be extended to weight loss diets for specific groups of people, like those with type 2 diabetes.[5] Basically, if different weight loss diets were racing, some of them do sprint out with a faster head start, but at the 12-month finish line, they all tend to cross at a similar time. What this means is you shouldn't really give two shits about which diet is best on paper, but instead find dietary approaches that suit your personal preferences. Some people like low-carb diets and some don't. Some people like eating a big breakfast and some don't. Some people like using meal replacement shakes and some don't. You get the idea.

This is absolutely critical to understand, because part of the reason people fall into the dreaded yo-yo dieting trap is because they follow a diet plan that they simply cannot adhere to in the long term. If you decide to start an ultra-low-carb keto diet today because someone twisted your arm into believing that it is the best diet for everyone, but your favorite foods are high in carbohydrates like pasta, bread, rice and potatoes, the likelihood of you sticking to that diet for years hovers dangerously close to absolutely zero. Although this is an extreme example, it epitomizes what tends to happen with all weight loss diets. People's adherence wanes over time and any initial success they achieved is often very short-lived. This is not a secret and it has been known for a long time. For example, one research study from 2005 tested four different weight loss diets to see which was most effective and, over the course of 12 months, the adherence rate of all of them started high and then dropped faster than the average home value during the great 2008 market crash.[6]

It is also important to remember that any dietary tips you follow should not be viewed solely by whether you lose weight or not. Too many people try to reduce their weight by any means necessary and at any cost. Losing weight is easy—just follow any reduced-calorie diet for a long enough period of time. Losing weight sustainably and keeping it off in the long term, while improving your health and without accidentally drop-kicking your mental health off a cliff, is where the real trophy needs to be. Your overall well-being is far more multifaceted than what the number on the scales says.

In this chapter, we are going to discuss the three broad categories that every fat loss diet tends to fall under—those that manipulate your macronutrient intake, those that tell you which foods to focus on or which ones to minimize and those that manipulate your meal timing. Importantly, these are not mutually exclusive. For example, some people might follow a low-carb diet, which is a macronutrient manipulation, but also do so in the context of a time-restricted feeding diet, which is a timing manipulation. While any of the following diets or eating plans may or may not work for you, what is most important is that you pair some or all of the behaviors that are discussed in Chapter 5—the 13 healthy habits—alongside your chosen eating regimen.

## Macronutrient-Based Diets

The three macronutrients are proteins, carbohydrates and fats, which give us energy and enable the body to carry out its essential functions. Different foods within each macronutrient group will then contain micronutrients like vitamins and minerals. We need macronutrients in larger amounts than micronutrients (hence "macro"), though some diets will prescribe a very specific macronutrient ratio, like "You absolutely must avoid all carbohydrates" or "You must cut back on fat as much as humanly possible." Many people get obsessive about what macronutrients they eat, but this often misses the forest for the trees, because the macronutrient content of your diet actually tells you very little about how nutritious it is.

For example, you could follow a low-fat diet by prioritizing lean proteins like chicken and white fish, eating plenty of fresh fruits and vegetables, and consuming more minimally processed carbohydrates like potatoes, rice and oatmeal. You could also maintain a low-fat diet by eating nothing but jellybeans and gummy worms and drinking sugary soda. Technically, both of these could be equally low in fat, but it doesn't take a genius to realize that they are not equally healthy. Similarly, you could reduce your carb intake by eating a diet full of nutritious foods like oily fish, lean meats, nuts and green vegetables— but still be following a low-carb diet when exclusively consuming deep-fried bacon, cheese and hot dogs, without the bun, of course. In addition, if you steer clear of whole food groups, this can increase your overall risk of nutrient deficiencies.

Following a specific macronutrient diet doesn't guarantee good nutritional quality overall or how you will feel while you're following that program, so people who hyperfocus on macronutrients and nothing else are often being silly sausages who miss the bigger picture.

### Low-carb diets

Carbohydrates are found in starchy foods like bread, pasta, oats, rice and potatoes, but are also found in sweet foods like fruit and honey (where the sugars are naturally occurring) and sodas, candy, cakes, cookies, and so on (where the sugars are normally refined and added into the product to improve the flavor).

Low-carb diets vary depending on how strictly you intend to avoid carbohydrates. Some diets just steer you away from obviously less nutritious refined carb-rich foods, like candy, sugary sodas, cakes, pastries, ice cream and doughnuts. Other diets, like very-low-carbohydrate ketogenic (keto) diets, are much more extreme and will tell you to dodge *all* significant sources of carbs, including bread, rice, pasta, oatmeal and potatoes. Popular branded weight loss plans that have a reduced carbohydrate intake include Atkins, South Beach, Dukan and Paleo.[7] Sometimes these are not branded as low-carb diets as such, but the foods they tell you to eat or avoid can nudge you toward eating fewer carbohydrates.

Fans of low-carb diets often claim that carbohydrates are uniquely fattening foods because they stimulate the hormone insulin, which will preferentially store the calories in that food in your body fat.[8] Food contains energy that you can store or burn off, and the energy within carbohydrates somehow gets an express train ticket straight into your body fat. The scientific theory has changed a bit over the years, like whether low-carb diets are better for appetite regulation, or whether specific carbohydrates like sugars are more fattening than starches, but that's the super-simple take-home message.[9,10]

A big plus side of low-carbohydrate diets is that people who follow them often lose body fat without having to do any kind of calorie counting.[11] Weighing everything you eat and calculating the calorie value of it is a chore that most people outside of hardcore fitness circles would rather not bother with, so following a diet plan that promises no calorie counting can be tempting. Low-carbohydrate and ketogenic diets may not officially tell you to restrict how many calories you consume,[12] but they may tell you the maximum number of carbohydrates you can eat per day (like 50g—or around 1.8oz—for example) or they will give you a list of foods you cannot eat. Another plus side for low-carbohydrate diets is that people who follow them also tend to consume more protein, and this can be good for promoting fat loss and muscle growth.[13,14]

Your body naturally stores carbohydrates (broken down into glucose in your body and stored as glycogen) and water, both of which are acutely influenced by how many carbs you are eating, so when you suddenly stop eating carbohydrates, it's common for your body weight to drop rapidly—but this does not necessarily mean you have lost body fat.[15] Going on a low-carb diet is a bit like squeezing water out of a sponge; the sponge gets lighter very quickly, but is also susceptible to regaining weight just as fast. Many low-carb dieters attest that their weight can shoot back up after just one high-carb meal and, once again, this is not always indicative of body fat changes. Short-term fluctuations in how much you weigh can be misleading when trying to work out what your body fat percentage actually is.

Just like hairstyles and funky clothing choices, diet plans tend to go in and out of fashion, and, at the time of writing, low-carbohydrate diets are very popular. However, restricting how many carbohydrates you eat is probably not better for losing body fat than restricting how much dietary fat you eat, unless one of them is better for regulating your appetite and causes you to eat fewer calories than the other.[16] Although some people love low-carb plans, they don't appear to be significantly easier for everyone to stick to in the long term.[17] Most people do not want to spend their life dodging sandwiches, let alone all cereal, pasta, rice and potatoes.

Basically, some of you like carbs, some of you are indifferent and some of you don't care for them. Although most people would benefit from eating less refined carbohydrate-rich foods, like candy, cakes, doughnuts, muffins and other delicious baked goods, it's unfortunately common for people to become unnecessarily carb-phobic. If you anxiously avoid a long list of foods that you enjoy and become too paranoid to let yourself eat a single apple, your diet is not a win regardless of what happens to your body fat percentage.

### Low-fat diets

These are effectively the reverse of the above, as low-fat diets tend to be high in carbohydrates and vice versa. After all, if you are told to limit foods that are high in dietary fats, you need to replace them with something else, and the remaining options are carbohydrates or protein. Several diets and nutritional approaches encourage you to reduce how much fat you eat, including the Ornish and Rosemary Conley methods,[18] as well as the Nordic Nutrition Recommendations, plant-based vegan diets and recommendations from institutions like the American Heart Association,[19] the National Health Service (NHS) in England and the WHO.

Dietary fat can be broken up into two broad categories: saturated and unsaturated fat:

- Saturated fat is typically solid at room temperature and naturally found in many animal products like red meat, butter, cheese and lard. A lot of dietary advice to limit fat intake is focused on saturated fat specifically, whereas unsaturated fats tend to be viewed as healthier, on average.

- Unsaturated fats tend to be liquid at room temperature and are further divided into:
    - Monounsaturated fats, which are found in olive oil, avocados, nuts and seeds, and some vegetable oils.
    - Polyunsaturated fats, which are often higher in oily fish like salmon and mackerel, but also some nuts, seeds and vegetable oils as well.
    - Trans fats. Although small amounts of trans fats can be naturally occurring, these are predominantly found in foods like partially hydrogenated oils, which are chemically altered liquid fats that are made to be solid at room temperature. Government agencies like the US Food and Drug Administration (FDA) have taken steps to minimize artificial trans fats in the food supply.

Although there are other subcategories, these are the most common terms you will see and they often coexist in foods. For example, avocados contain saturated, monounsaturated and polyunsaturated fat, but much higher levels of monounsaturated fat, specifically. Dietary fat has more calories per gram than carbohydrates and protein (9 calories per gram for fat versus 4 calories per gram for carbohydrates and protein), so, in theory, reducing dietary fat is a super-easy way to reduce your calorie intake. If you have a plateful of higher-fat foods like steak cooked in butter or scrambled eggs with cheese and bacon, this will be higher in calories than a plate that weighs exactly the same but contains lower-fat foods like grilled chicken, rice and vegetables. This is because higher-fat foods have a greater "energy density," meaning more calories per gram of food. So, prioritizing lower-fat foods actually makes sense for appetite regulation because you can eat a higher quantity of food for the same number of calories.[20] In theory, you could keep all of your food choices very similar but swap them for lower-fat options and lose body fat,[21,22] which is one reason why low-fat diets used to be extremely popular.

Just like low-carb diets, low-fat diets can vary in how extreme they are. Some recommendations are actually the same as low-carb programs, because limiting calorie-dense ultra-processed foods that are high in fats and sugars (like cookies, doughnuts and ice cream) is a smart idea regardless of what diet you follow. Some low-fat guidelines are quite gentle, like trimming excess fat off red meat, removing the skin from chicken, opting for lower-fat dairy options and limiting how much fat you cook with—for example, swapping frying and deep-frying for grilling and air-frying. Other recommendations are much more extreme, like avoiding all red meat in favor of white meat, removing the egg yolks in favor of only eating egg whites and limiting *any* added fats, like cooking oils and butter.

As with low-carb diets, it's quite possible to lose body fat on a low-fat diet without proactively counting calories. While that is definitely a bonus on paper, it's probably largely because diets that severely restrict your food choices make it harder to overeat. If you are told that you can't eat any high-calorie ultra-processed foods, deep-fried foods, fatty red meats, high-fat dairy or additional cooking oils, then it is inevitable you will be pushed toward lower-calorie food choices. While low-fat diets are not associated with the same rapid *weight* loss that low-carb diets tend to have, the actual *fat* loss you can achieve on low-fat diets is very similar.[23]

Basically, what this means is that both low-carb and low-fat diets can help you to consume fewer calories, which appears to be the most important factor in whether you lose body fat, not some elusive macronutrient ratio, like many people claim.[24] Neither option is magic, and whether you have success with them depends entirely on whether you can stick with them in the long term. Think of it like worrying about whether running or cycling is better for improving your fitness levels. While some people seem hell-bent on arguing the merits of each, I personally think this is a massive waste of time. Instead, rest assured knowing that you can get great health benefits from either, if you 1) have a nutritious dietary pattern, 2) consume an appropriate number of calories for your goal, and 3) do them consistently for a long period of time, so it makes more sense to just pick what you enjoy, even if that's different from what your friend enjoys.

### A final note on low-carb and low-fat diets

Macronutrient-based weight loss diets often impose intense food restrictions as a way to force you to decrease your calorie intake, which is why some low-carb diet plans tell you to consume fewer than 50g (1.8oz) of carbohydrates per day, or some low-fat plans tell you to aim for fewer than 15 percent of your calories from fat. Both of these can be difficult targets to achieve without completely overhauling what you eat. Although we have examined the polar ends of the spectrum, there are obviously many more moderate, balanced macronutrient diets in the middle, including The Biggest Loser, Mediterranean, DASH, Jenny Craig, Weight Watchers and Slimming World.[25]

By understanding the macronutrient diet spectrum, why different diets work and how they work, you can also understand why it might be a smarter idea for you to avoid diets that sound unworkable for you. For example, if you really love eating rice, pasta and bread, a low-carb diet sounds like an absolute nightmare, but if you also love eating red meat, avocados and butter, a low-fat diet might be just as horrific and equally difficult to achieve. One thing that both of these approaches agree upon is that decreasing your intake of extremely calorie-dense ultra-processed foods, like chocolate, cookies and cake, is a good idea. Perhaps a more balanced approach might tickle your fancy instead.

### High-protein diets

Protein gets a lot of love for its role in muscle building and recovery. If you go to a public gym, chances are you will see a whole array of protein powders, drinks and bars lining the shelves. Historically, these have been aimed at the niche subgroup of gym dudes trying to bulk up and get buff, and they would have ridiculous names like "Extreme Muscle Growth XXXL 5000," but, more recently, protein products have diversified and also become popular with women and with people trying to lose body fat rather than just build muscle. Gone are the days of steroid-fueled bodybuilders appearing on the front of protein powder tubs. The mainstream appeal means we now also get protein powder in pink packaging, using words like "lean protein," "shaping" and "toning."

This is because high-protein diets may also be useful from a weight and fat loss perspective.[26,27] If you lose a lot of weight, it is common to lose some muscle tissue in the process, but consuming more protein can help mitigate this.[28] This is a good thing. After all, if you lose a lot of weight, you probably don't want a big chunk of that to be muscle mass, right? Even if you don't give a shit how you look in the mirror and have no desire to have a visibly muscular or toned physique, muscle mass can help keep you strong and increase your longevity when aging starts taking its toll on your strength, mobility and quality of life.[29] When dieting, having more muscle can also play a small role in keeping your metabolic rate high (the amount of energy you burn per day), and consuming more protein can help with appetite regulation.[30] Some protein-rich foods are probably good for helping you feel full,[31] and that is always welcome when dieting because being hungry all the time is a miserable way to live. That being said, some people probably worship high-protein diets a little too much, because it's not as simple as saying, "Eat more protein and you will definitely feel less hungry."

If you are losing weight and consuming enough protein to hold on to muscle mass, the remaining ratio of carbohydrates to fat is probably not worth worrying about.[32] People can get super obsessive about what their macronutrient ratios are, like trying to eat 40 percent protein, 40 percent carbohydrates and 20 percent fat. In reality, if you are getting enough protein to maintain that precious muscle tissue when dieting, you can fill your remaining calorie allowance with whatever foods suit your personal preference, because the difference it makes is probably half a smidge above absolutely fuck all. It is not worth trying to follow a very specific macronutrient plan if that involves sacrificing your ability to stick with it.

## Predominant Macronutrient Content of Some Example Popular Foods

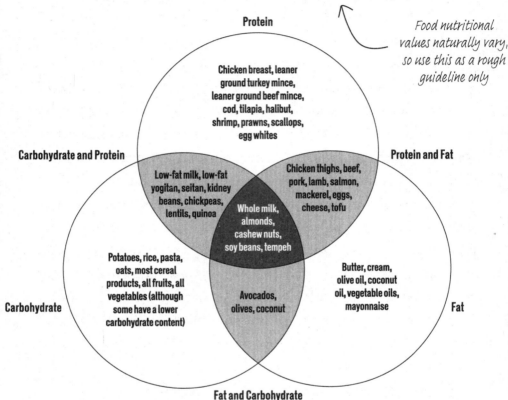

Food nutritional values naturally vary, so use this as a rough guideline only

Protein

Chicken breast, leaner ground turkey mince, leaner ground beef mince, cod, tilapia, halibut, shrimp, prawns, scallops, egg whites

Carbohydrate and Protein

Protein and Fat

Low-fat milk, low-fat yogitan, seitan, kidney beans, chickpeas, lentils, quinoa

Chicken thighs, beef, pork, lamb, salmon, mackerel, eggs, cheese, tofu

Whole milk, almonds, cashew nuts, soy beans, tempeh

Potatoes, rice, pasta, oats, most cereal products, all fruits, all vegetables (although some have a lower carbohydrate content)

Avocados, olives, coconut

Butter, cream, olive oil, coconut oil, vegetable oils, mayonnaise

Carbohydrate

Fat

Fat and Carbohydrate

## Food-Choice Diets

Rather than searching for a magical macronutrient ratio, many diets prefer to tell you which foods to prioritize or which to limit. These programs are often less extreme than diets that say you are never allowed to lick an apple again because it's too high in carbohydrates, or you are never allowed to even look at a steak again because it's too high in saturated fat. By focusing on foods that are nutritious, and often good for regulating your appetite, food-choice diets can also teach us some useful weight-management lessons. Let's talk about some of the most popular ones.

### The Mediterranean diet

This is not a weight loss diet as such, but instead is well recognized as being one of the healthiest dietary patterns in the world.[33] It is very difficult to study the long-term health effects of any diet, because you can't exactly lock a thousand people into a research facility for 70 years, give half of the group a Mediterranean diet and see how many of them get heart disease, cancer or die compared to the other half of the group. That kind of study probably wouldn't be approved for ethical reasons, obviously. However, based on the available research we have, the Mediterranean diet appears to be associated with improvements for a whole shitload of different medical concerns, including risk factors of metabolic syndrome, some cancers, cardiovascular diseases, coronary heart disease and type 2 diabetes.[34,35] Not only that, but eating a Mediterranean diet is linked with a decreased risk of all-cause mortality.[36] Basically, people who more closely adhere to a Mediterranean diet appear to be healthier and also live a bit longer, which is a big yay. This is especially emphasized in people who live in Mediterranean regions, perhaps because their diets tend to be especially high in olive oil, fish, vegetables and legumes, but also possibly because of other lifestyle factors.

Although there isn't a very firm definition of what a Mediterranean diet is, it is typically higher in fish, legumes, fruits, vegetables, wholegrains, nuts and olive oil, with a moderate intake of wine and sometimes lower amounts of red meats, processed meats and dairy products.[37] Generally speaking, these are nutritious foods, right? A Mediterranean dietary pattern tends to be rich in fiber, monounsaturated and polyunsaturated fats plus vitamins, minerals, polyphenols and phytosterols, which are compounds naturally found in plants that are linked with health benefits. It's not a diet that is high in hot dogs, bacon, double cheeseburgers and doughnuts. Diets high in nutrient-dense unprocessed foods tend to have a lower energy density and therefore also tend to be better for regulating your appetite and making you feel full, and when your appetite is lower you tend to eat fewer calories and lose weight.[38]

I imagine precisely zero people on the planet start the Mediterranean diet with the sole goal of having a shredded six-pack, and it lacks the flashy marketing campaigns and expensive advertising budgets that many branded diet plans have. This means it rarely gets a mention when people argue about the best weight loss diets, but some research does show that it can be used for fat loss purposes, when combined with a reduced calorie intake, of course.[39]

It might not be the best diet for losing body fat (given there is no universally *best* diet for losing body fat), but that is like judging how useful your favorite pet dog is by its ability to fly or how valuable your parents are by their ability to time travel. That's just not the thing they are supposed to be best at, so don't judge them by that metric. You can technically combine any dietary pattern with an increase or decrease in your calorie consumption, so if you do plan on reducing your calorie intake to lose body fat, why not do so with a unanimously agreed health-promoting dietary pattern?

## The DASH diet

DASH stands for "Dietary Approaches to Stop Hypertension." This obviously isn't the coolest sounding name, so it makes sense that they use a catchy acronym. "Hypertension" is just a fancier word for "high blood pressure," so, just like the Mediterranean diet, the DASH diet is largely judged on whether it can improve your health, rather than whether it can decrease your waistline. The DASH diet has been funded by the US National Heart, Lung and Blood Institute (NHLBI) for around three decades now and its original objective was to tackle the worrying prevalence of high blood pressure in America, which was estimated to affect 24 percent of American adults at the time.[40] High blood pressure is well known to be a leading cause of an alarming number of deaths around the world[41] and, while medication can obviously be used to treat this, it would also be delightful if people could implement dietary and lifestyle changes that would reduce their risk of something catastrophic happening to their health.[42]

Although it's not really marketed as a weight loss diet as such, the first dietary trials did note that obesity is a risk factor for high blood pressure, so, with the goal of improving your health, it is quite possible that, if you follow the diet, you will also lose weight.[43] If you want, you can view weight loss as the sometimes-welcome side effect of a healthy nutritional pattern, rather than as the sole focus. There have been several research trials on the DASH diet[44,45,46,47] and although its dietary recommendations might vary a tad, the general vibe is that this diet is rich in fruits, vegetables, wholegrains, legumes, low-fat dairy foods, fish, poultry, nuts, seeds and vegetable oils. You would also limit your intake of fatty red meat, full-fat dairy, sugary drinks and sweets to help reduce your intake of saturated fat and added sugars. Specific to the DASH diet is regulating your sodium—or salt—intake and having a diet rich in potassium, for blood pressure purposes specifically.

As DASH diets are not trying to be sexy, highly marketed rapid weight loss diets, their research studies just tend to compare variations of the DASH diet to a standard diet. This shows that if you are eating a typical Western diet, high in calories, saturated fats, added sugars and salt, and low in fresh produce like fruits and vegetables, like a lot of people in America and other countries are, and you switch to the DASH diet, then you will probably lose weight and improve your health. This is a bit like comparing running to sitting on the couch. Of course, running is better for your health, but it doesn't necessarily mean running is better than cycling, swimming or rowing. It just means that running is definitely better than doing absolutely jack shit. Basically, the DASH diet is not fighting among other aggressive weight loss diets to see which deserves the crown for reducing your waistline the fastest. It is, very simply, a nutritious dietary pattern that often tips you toward losing weight, especially if you deliberately try to reduce your calorie intake at the same time.[48]

### The Paleo diet

Paleo is short for "Paleolithic" and is also known as the "caveman diet." It is high in vegetables, fruits, meat, eggs and nuts, which means it actually has a sizable overlap with the Mediterranean and DASH diets. The basic premise of this is very simple. A lot of the tasty treats we are surrounded by nowadays are manufactured by big food companies and didn't exist hundreds of years ago, let alone thousands or millions of years ago, so if we revert to only eating foods that were available to cavemen, we might escape some of the diseases that appear to be more prevalent now than they used to be, including obesity.[49] What did cavemen not eat? Well, they definitely didn't eat cakes, cookies, doughnuts, ice cream or chocolates. They didn't lie on the sofa binge-watching their favorite TV series and ordering takeout to be delivered to their door. So maybe reverting to our ancestral diet *would* be a smart idea?

If you choose to follow the Paleo diet, you would clearly have to cut out delicious high-calorie ultra-processed foods as these weren't available to cavemen. You would exclude alcohol, refined sugars and refined oils like vegetable oil, too. However, the more contentious aspect of Paleo is that you would also have to avoid some standard staples like all grains, dairy and sometimes even potatoes and added salt, which is a pretty hefty restriction to then stack on top.[50] The reason this gets controversial is because we know these foods can fit into other nutritious dietary patterns, like the Mediterranean diet and the DASH diet that we have discussed already. So, is it really necessary to avoid these common food types as well? As with diets that focus on a specific macronutrient, if you have to steer clear of several whole food groups, isn't that increasing your risk of nutrient deficiencies, ultimately making the diet plan far more painful than it is worth? Some diets fall down the slippery slope of being unnecessarily restrictive, to the point they can make you terrified of eating perfectly acceptable foods. This can make plans like the Paleo diet very hard for you to stick with in the long term. Rather laughably, one research study described the Paleo diet as "impractical for use in public health settings."[51] In other words, following this diet can be so difficult that prescribing it to big groups of people might be a recipe for disaster.

The extreme avoidance of so many food groups, plus prioritizing unprocessed foods, which tend to be better for appetite regulation,[52] is quite a potent combination for forcing you to reduce how many calories you consume. Therefore, it comes as no surprise that people who follow the Paleo diet do seem to lose weight and often improve their health markers in the process,[53,54,55] even if they do not consistently get much better results than those following Mediterranean or DASH diets.[56]

Long story short, while the Paleo diet can definitely work if you want to lose weight and improve your health, the extreme restrictions make it tougher to adhere to than most people would like. Dieting can sometimes feel hard, like walking a tightrope. The Paleo diet is like choosing to cross that same tightrope on a unicycle. It's making things significantly more difficult (unless you just so happen to be someone who is really proficient at unicycling).

### Plant-based diets

Most people who follow plant-based diets do not jump into them because they have a beach holiday coming up and they suddenly want to try to get a six-pack. Instead, they tend to be diets that people adopt for health or ethical reasons, like vegans completely abstaining from consuming animal products. To some vegans, calling veganism a "diet" is actually offensive because it implies they are just hopping on another fad diet, rather than choosing to minimize animal cruelty as a way of life. However, the word "diet" also just means what you eat, and plant-based diets are becoming more popular among the health-conscious crowd as well, so let's briefly discuss what we know for sure.

"Plant-based" is actually a big umbrella term for lots of different dietary approaches. At one end of the spectrum, you have vegans who avoid consuming all animal-based foods. Covering the rest of the spectrum you have vegetarians whose diets can vary a lot. Depending on the type of vegetarianism, like lacto-vegetarianism, ovo-vegetarianism, lacto-ovo-vegetarianism and pesco-vegetarianism, they might avoid eating meat but still consume dairy; eggs; dairy and eggs; or fish, dairy and eggs, in some combination. You also have some people who describe themselves as "plant-based" but still consume some animal products very sporadically. This makes it tricky to discuss them all without waffling on for pages and pages, so the simplified summary notes are: the fewer animal products people eat, the more plant products they tend to eat to fill the gap. This doesn't automatically make a diet healthier because yes, fruits and vegetables are obviously suitable for vegans, but you can also buy vegan doughnuts and vegan cookies, plus vegan pizzas, vegan burgers and vegan sausages, which can sometimes contain as much added sugar and fat as their non-vegan counterparts, so the absence of animal products tells us very little about whether plant-based diets are guaranteed to be healthier.

As people who follow plant-based diets often do tend to be more health-conscious, your average vegetarian is likely to smoke less, drink less alcohol and be more physically active than your average meat-eater.[57] They often have a reduced risk of many health conditions, including type 2 diabetes, ischemic heart disease, some types of cancer and obesity.[58] But understanding all the pros and cons of vegetarian diets is actually quite a pickle. If your average vegetarian is healthier than your average meat-eater, is it because eating meat and fish is dangerous? Or is it because they tend to consume more fruits, vegetables, wholegrains and legumes,[59] which are foods that overlap with other healthy dietary patterns we have already discussed? One thing that we can say with quite a high degree of certainty is that eating more fruits, vegetables, wholegrains and legumes often has the added effect of helping people to consume fewer calories as these are foods with more fiber and a lower energy density, and when people eat fewer calories and lose weight, some health markers often improve.[60] There is actually quite a lot of research showing that vegetarian and vegan diets promote weight loss and improved health.[61,62]

Does it mean they are risk-free, though? Absolutely not. Vegan diets often need to be supplemented with vitamin B12 for example,[63] and there might be a heightened risk of other nutrient deficiencies.[64] Vegetarians often consume a little less protein than meat-eaters and, given that protein is important for muscle recovery, this in theory could make them more likely to lose muscle tissue while they are following a plant-based diet, but some research studies just overcome this hurdle by giving the participants more protein powder.[65] Although there are possible drawbacks of plant-based diets, as most people who follow them decide to do it for ethical or health reasons, spending too much time obsessing over whether they are best for losing body fat would be focusing too much attention on the wrong thing.

### A final note on food-choice diets

There are many other popular diets I could list in this section, but I just wanted to give you a quick and dirty lowdown of the most common ones. Although they sound very different, the eagle-eyed among you will have probably noticed a common theme. Mediterranean, DASH, Paleo and plant-based diets actually all seem to have something in common. They recommend decreasing your intake of ultra-processed foods that are high in calories, added sugars and added fats, and encourage eating more nutrient-dense unprocessed foods. Sure, some of these vary a bit, like you can eat fish on a Mediterranean diet but not on some plant-based diets, or you can eat wholegrains on the DASH diet but not on the Paleo diet. But overall, they all tend to agree that eating more fruits, vegetables and nuts is a good idea. The remaining gray areas revolve around how many grains you should eat (like rice, bread and pasta), whether you should eat lean meat or fattier cuts of red meat (not applicable to vegetarian and vegan diets, obviously), and how liberally you should use added butter and oils, if at all.

One of the most important things I would like you to take from this section is that measuring a diet based on how many calories you eat or what macronutrients you prefer fails to take into account the quality of the food you are eating and how nutritious your overall diet is. Health-promoting diets often don't give many fucks about people trying to do silly things like lose 4.5kg (10lb) in a week, but instead place more emphasis on overall dietary patterns that can improve your well-being. In a world full of aggressive crash diets that often make you feel like you are permanently restricting and avoiding, focusing more on the nutritious foods you *can* eat in abundance can feel like a refreshing change. Following a healthy dietary pattern, such as the Mediterranean or DASH diet, without the accompanying calorie restriction might not get you to lose weight as rapidly as any very-low-calorie crash diet will, but if you manage to create sustainable dietary habits you can stick to, you might actually end up in a better place anyway.

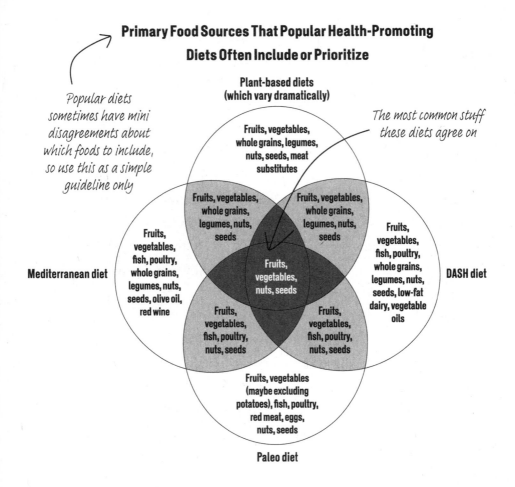

Primary Food Sources That Popular Health-Promoting Diets Often Include or Prioritize

*Popular diets sometimes have mini disagreements about which foods to include, so use this as a simple guideline only*

**Plant-based diets** (which vary dramatically)

*The most common stuff these diets agree on*

Fruits, vegetables, whole grains, legumes, nuts, seeds, meat substitutes

Fruits, vegetables, whole grains, legumes, nuts, seeds

Fruits, vegetables, whole grains, legumes, nuts, seeds

**Mediterranean diet**

Fruits, vegetables, fish, poultry, whole grains, legumes, nuts, seeds, olive oil, red wine

Fruits, vegetables, nuts, seeds

**DASH diet**

Fruits, vegetables, fish, poultry, whole grains, legumes, nuts, seeds, low-fat dairy, vegetable oils

Fruits, vegetables, fish, poultry, nuts, seeds

Fruits, vegetables, fish, poultry, nuts, seeds

Fruits, vegetables (maybe excluding potatoes), fish, poultry, red meat, eggs, nuts, seeds

**Paleo diet**

## Meal-Timing Diets

We now come to the third big umbrella group of diets, which are based not on what macronutrients or foods you eat, but on what time you eat them.

Meal-timing diets are entirely different from the macronutrient-based diets and food-choice diets above as they tell you absolutely zero about the macronutrients or foods you choose to prioritize. They very simply tell you *when* you should or shouldn't eat, and that's about it. The following diets—the 16:8 diet, alternate-day fasting and the 5:2 diet—all fall under the umbrella of fasting diets. Their other common names are time-restricted feeding or time-restricted eating, intermittent fasting or intermittent energy restriction, and their popularity has grown rapidly in the past decade or so.

### Time-restricted feeding

For a long time, people have argued about whether breakfast is the most important meal of the day. Some people say you need to eat a big breakfast because it helps "kick-start your metabolism" or some shit like that—an idea that just doesn't make sense. Your metabolism basically refers to the sum of all chemical processes in your body.[66] If your metabolism has stopped, it means you are dead and you have bigger problems to worry about than whether you should eat breakfast. Your metabolism is not a lawn mower you have to crank every time you want to get it going. It is always going because you are alive.

Time-restricted feeding plans are in some ways the opposite of this pro-breakfast advice, because they specifically focus on what periods of time you *shouldn't* eat.

Fasting is a very common religious practice. For example, Muslims fast during Ramadan and abstain from eating and drinking anything from sunrise to sunset. This Islamic tradition is not adopted by people because they are trying to get a six-pack, and that is precisely why it teaches us some valuable lessons. When Muslims abstain from eating food for long periods of time during Ramadan, it is quite common for them to lose some weight, including body fat.[67] This can also occur in tandem with improvements in health markers like blood glucose, cholesterol and blood pressure.[68]

Basically, if you tell people to avoid food for long periods of time, guess what happens? Drumroll, please...They tend to eat less food. I know that sounds like I am pointing out the blatantly fucking obvious, but a lot of people seem surprisingly confused about how and why time-restricted feeding works.

So, take this basic principle and apply it to common weight loss diets. The most well-known time-restricted feeding diet is called 16:8, where you abstain from eating food for 16 hours of each day and you only eat food in the remaining 8 hours.[69] If you eat lunch and dinner between the hours of midday and 8pm and eat nothing else outside of those hours, you are doing a form of fasting known as a time-restricted feeding diet. Coincidentally, do you know what else this can be referred to as? Skipping breakfast.

If you tell people to skip breakfast, it is quite common that they will finish the day having eaten less food, so just the simple act of breakfast skipping can often promote a teeny bit of weight loss even if you don't bother giving them any more specific dietary advice.[70] But, it's also possible that something else happens. If I tell you to skip breakfast, your appetite might increase, so when lunch and dinner finally come around you are ready to devour not just your regular meals, but also the entire contents of your snack cupboard. Alternatively, you skip breakfast but don't even make it to lunch because you spend your whole morning feeling exponentially more snack-curious, so you tuck into the doughnuts kept at the office. While telling people to skip a meal might make sense in helping to reduce their calorie intake, it can also accidentally backfire if their appetite increases to compensate for that deprivation, which could be a reason why some people who skip breakfast actually tend to weigh more than those who eat it.[71] Skipping meals only works reliably for weight loss if you don't get hungrier and eat more at your next meal or resort to extra snacking, and that is a gigantic "if."

So here is the big debate. Let's say you start doing 16:8 time-restricted feeding and, after a few weeks, you notice you have lost some body fat and you are feeling a bit healthier. This is obviously great news. But does this mean there is something magical about that 16-hour fasting window? Or did you simply skip a meal you eat regularly, eat less food overall and lose weight, which caused your health markers to improve? A lot of people are overselling the shit out of fasting diets and making it sound like they are the secret key to optimal health, happiness and longevity, but the benefits always appear to be more prevalent when it causes someone to eat less food. When comparing time-restricted feeding to a regular reduced-calorie diet with the same amount of food, it seems a lot of the benefits suddenly vanish into thin air.[72,73] For example, in one study the researchers decided to do something extra meticulous and actually provide all the food for the participants, ensuring that the total number of calories and macronutrient breakdown was precisely weighed and exactly the same, with one exception: one group consumed their meals in a ten-hour feeding window and the other group could eat their meals whenever they wanted.[74] When the two diets were exactly the same, what extra weight loss benefits did the fasting window provide? Zero.

## When Does Time-Restricted Eating Work?

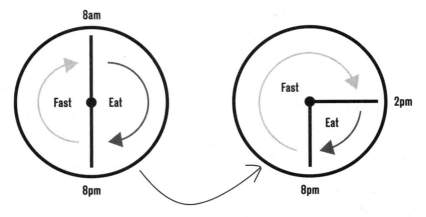

*Switching from this to this often causes people to eat fewer calories without even realizing it, which promotes weight loss and can improve some health markers. But in research studies where the calorie intake is kept the same, the weight loss benefits seem to disappear.*

It is totally true that fasting can improve many people's health. But whether you actually need to avoid food for long periods of time to obtain all those health benefits is an ongoing debate. It's possible that fasting could improve some health markers even if you don't eat less,[75] but, at the moment, solely from a weight loss perspective, I think it's sensible to play it safe and just view it as a tool that often nudges people toward eating less food.

One big plus point of time-restricted feeding is that it is simple, because saying, "Hey, don't eat breakfast" or "Only eat between midday and 8pm" is dietary advice that takes literally five seconds to tell someone and, occasionally, that sound bite alone is enough to promote weight loss. Another possible advantage is that people who adopt this kind of fasting protocol often find themselves eating fewer calories than they would on a normal diet, which can give them a little extra weight loss edge.[76] That said, if they are going to eat exactly the same amount of food and just squish it into a smaller time frame, it's probably not going to do a lot.[77]

A big negative of this kind of diet is that, if avoiding food for longer periods of time makes you want to eat more in the hours you aren't fasting, your body might feel inclined to scarf down food at a faster rate to make up for what you missed out on. From a weight loss perspective, this is like taking two steps forward and another two back again. From a psychological perspective, it can trigger many more steps backward if you find yourself slipping into the dangerous habit of binge eating in the evenings, which is a legitimate concern.[78] In my opinion, it is extremely irresponsible that so many intermittent fasting proponents do not seem to acknowledge this as a risk. If you lose a few pounds but your relationship with food is atrocious and you feel like you cycle between overly restricting what you eat and engaging in subsequent uncontrollable binge eating, that is not a win.

### Alternate-day fasting

OK, so we know that if we tell people to avoid food for a big chunk of the day, they tend to eat less food. No surprises there. Let's take that principle and extend it out over the course of the week. Rather than saying, "Hey, why don't you skip breakfast and eat all your food in an eight-hour window?," alternate-day fasting is basically saying, "If you eat absolutely no food, or heavily restrict what you eat, every other day of the week, you can probably eat whatever you want on the remaining days."

Think of it like this: let's say you have an exam coming up and you need to study hard for it. One obvious option is to do some reviewing every single day. But some people might find that frustratingly painful, like peeling a Band-Aid off incredibly slowly. Are you dragging out the discomfort for longer than necessary? After all, if you are studying daily, then it interferes with the rest of your life every single day as well. A different method is to cram all your reviewing into a few days of the week and do absolutely zero reviewing on the other days. Yes, the studying days are more grueling, but if you work really hard on those days then you can chill out on the others. Look at it like an intense part-time schedule, where you are working overtime for three to four days a week and then resting completely on the days in between. That's the basic idea of alternate-day fasting.

We know that sticking to a calorie-controlled diet every day is difficult, so wouldn't it be easier if you just did it less frequently? In 2005, one of the first research papers testing this in humans described alternate-day fasting as a "less complicated method" of losing weight than reducing your calorie intake by a little bit every single day.[79] In theory, if you reduce your food intake by an extreme amount on some days, maybe you can get away with eating whatever you want on the remaining days and still lose weight? As it turns out, yes. All you need to do is tell people to avoid food completely (zero-calorie alternate-day fasting) or really aggressively cut down what they eat (modified alternate-day fasting) on alternating days of the week, and that prescription alone is enough to promote weight loss even if you let people eat whatever the fuck they want on the other days.[80,81,82]

Although this sounds like it could be promising as an alternative weight loss strategy, I think we need to address the elephant in the room. While the idea of eating whatever you want on some days of the week might sound appealing, eating nothing, or very close to nothing, on alternating days of the week is not something many people fancy doing. For example, one early research trial lasting a mere 22 days said that many of the participants felt irritable on their fasting days, and to quote the study directly, "perhaps indicating the unlikelihood of continuing this diet for extended periods of time."[83] Personally, I would rather floss my teeth with a stranger's pubic hair than go entire days without eating anything. But it's important to remember that, if this kind of diet sounds extreme, it is because a lot of people are desperate to lose weight and have struggled with many other diets in the past.

You can see the attraction of zero-calorie alternate-day fasting: it is so easy to prescribe. As with other intermittent fasting plans, you don't have to waste time counting your calories. You aren't given long lists of foods you can and can't eat. You aren't given any complicated advice at all. You can literally just be told "Don't eat anything every other day," and that's that. If dieting was a surgical procedure, calorie counting is like a precision laser that can take more time and effort but allows you to meticulously remove whatever you want. Alternate-day fasting is more like a rusty axe. It can get the job done but it's silly to pretend it isn't a bit fucking brutal.

A final downside to alternate-day fasting is, although it is a super-simple way to get people to eat less, if you actually compare it to an equivalent food intake spread across the week, the weight loss results often seem remarkably similar.[84] For example, one 12-month research study tested a 6-month weight loss phase and a 6-month weight-maintenance phase in the form of either alternate-day fasting or a regular old reduced-calorie diet and guess what happened? When both groups had the equivalent degree of calorie restriction, the fasting group didn't see superior body composition or health benefits.[85]

Returning to our exam studying analogy, if you cram 14 hours of studying into alternating days of the week, you probably won't get better results than just doing 2 hours per day because the total at the end of the week is still the same. Also, although alternate-day fasting can improve people's health, it seems that the vehicle it achieves this by is simply reducing how much you eat. If you eat exactly the same amount of food you normally would but squeeze it into alternating days, you are very unlikely to notice any weight loss or improved health markers.[86] The basic take-home message here? Alternate-day fasting is another way to reduce your food intake, but anyone who pretends it is magic for fat loss is probably pissing on your leg and telling you it is raining.

### The 5:2 diet

This became very popular because it was featured in several diet books. You might see phrases like "fast for two days, feast for five days," which sounds quite appealing, because the word "feast" doesn't appear in many diet books, and what better way to attract people than by implying they can eat more for five whole days out of every seven?

This is essentially a very close sibling to alternate-day fasting. Rather than avoiding food completely, or severely limiting what you eat on alternating days of the week, with the 5:2 diet you would just do it on two days of the week instead. Hypothetically, instead of reducing your calorie intake by 10–20 percent every day, you would reduce it by a whopping 75 percent on two days of the week and then do whatever you want on the other days. Using the studying analogy, instead of doing a bit of reviewing every single day, you would cram it all into two days of the week, but then take five whole days off. Whether this sounds appealing or not is down to your personal preference, I guess.

We already know that this kind of intermittent fasting diet can work from a weight loss perspective. The real question is, does it work better than regular dieting? As it turns out, probably not. Several research studies have tested 5:2 intermittent fasting against a regular dietary pattern where food is reduced a little bit each day, and the weight loss results come out pretty much the same.[87,88,89,90] Basically, this is yet another weight loss plan that might be marketed to you as better than all the rest, but it's probably just another tool in the toolbox—arguably no better or worse than boring old regular dieting where people eat slightly fewer calories every single day. Some of you might find intermittent fasting plans like the 5:2 diet better for appetite regulation, which could be a bonus. Maybe some of you find it easier to stick with in the long term, which again would be a bonus. But anyone who is selling you the 5:2 plan and acting like it is the magical weight loss solution for everyone is talking utter nonsense. For example, in one study where the weight loss results were similar, a higher percentage of the 5:2 diet participants complained of hunger (15 percent versus 0 percent), other negative physical symptoms like headaches, constipation and feeling cold (8 percent versus 0 percent) and difficulties fitting the diet into their daily routine (51 percent versus 30 percent).[91]

Ultimately, it looks like it is just another vehicle that takes you to the same destination as any reduced-calorie diet. Just be careful that going through long periods of avoiding food doesn't lead you to overcompensate on your feeding days. One study noted that people on the 5:2 diet ate significantly more food on the days immediately after their fasting days;[92] for example, eating significantly less food on Monday and Thursday, but then compensating by eating a lot more on Tuesday and Friday. From a weight loss perspective, this is a bit like pushing and pulling at the same time.

## When Does Intermittent Fasting Work?

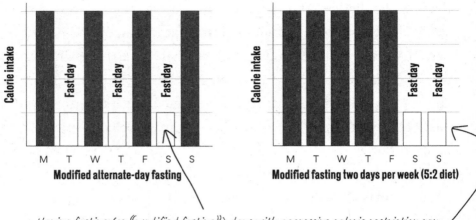

*Having fasting (or "modified fasting") days with aggressive calorie restriction can cause people to eat fewer total calories over the course of a week. But again, in newer research trials where they compare this to an equivalent degree of weekly calorie restriction via regular dieting, the weight loss and health benefits seem to vanish.*

It is true that meal-timing diets can promote weight loss and it is also true that these can often improve certain health markers. Whether they are better than traditional diets is a nerdy ongoing nutrition debate with people arguing from both sides, so there definitely isn't a super clear winner yet.[93,94,95] In my opinion, it is important for you to know this because it means you get to choose whichever approach floats your boat. If you prefer to avoid intermittent fasting, you can rest assured knowing it's not necessary to avoid food for long periods of time to lose body fat and improve your health.

The rising popularity of fasting diets unfortunately also means a lot of people exaggerate the shit out of their benefits, often in an attempt to sell you something that is pretty and shiny. Obviously, everything has pros and cons, and it concerns me that so many people selling time-restricted eating or intermittent fasting diets conveniently forget to tell you the downsides. Imagine you are a zookeeper looking after a tiger. Normally, it has a certain feeding schedule and, between those feeding times, it just lives its life, doing whatever tigers like to do. What happens if you put that tiger in a cage and stop feeding it? It is obviously going to get hungrier and hungrier, right? The longer it goes without eating, the more it starts thinking about food and the more food-obsessed it gets. At some point, it will get so ravenous that, when you finally let it out, it is going to hunt with far more desperation than it did before. Do you know what the difference is between you and a tiger in a zoo? Apart from the fact that it's an animal and you are a human, obviously. Well, you have far easier access to food. If you are hungry as fuck, you don't have to wait for a zookeeper to feed you. You just go to your fridge, pantry, snack cupboard or local grocery store and eat whatever you fancy. This is why fasting studies often highlight the risks of "overconsumption" during your feeding window, which is just a fancy term for depriving yourself of food for so long that you naturally want to stuff your face as soon as you can.

In its mildest form, you might eat slightly more food during your feeding window or feeding day than you would normally. At its most extreme, it could push you into a cycle of restricting yourself and then binge eating. There is a lack of research concretely confirming the link between fasting diets and eating disorders,[96] but it is an emerging topic that has sometimes been overly neglected,[97,98,99,100] with one recent research paper acknowledging that these diets might have therapeutic use, but this needs to be weighed up in a risk-to-reward fashion: "An important risk that intermittent fasting may pose is the potential to increase risk of disordered eating, which has only recently started to be examined."[101]

Nothing in this book should be perceived as personalized

medical information and eating disorders are a topic best reserved for specialists, but why don't more people selling fasting plans bother mentioning this to you? Ranking diets based solely on which promotes the most weight loss is actually quite short-sighted because many people try to lose weight via a method that sometimes comes with an extraordinarily high price tag, and that is a pitfall I would like to make sure you don't fall into from this point onward.

## How Popular Fat Loss Diets Really Work

| Nutrition Intervention | How Some People Think They Work | The Primary Reason They Actually Work |
|---|---|---|
| Low-carbohydrate diets | Carbohydrates are uniquely fattening; decreasing your intake lowers insulin production and promotes fat loss | Restricting carbs normally means people prioritize protein and eat fewer calories |
| Very-low-carbohydrate ketogenic diets | Going into a state called ketosis makes your body burn body fat at an accelerated rate | Strictly avoiding carbs often means people eat even more protein and even fewer calories than regular low-carb diets |
| Low-fat diets | By avoiding higher-fat foods, you can eat as much as you want of lower-fat foods and still lose weight | As dietary fat is calorie dense, reducing your intake is a fairly reliable, but not foolproof, way to reduce your calorie intake |
| Time-restricted feeding (16:8) diets | The long fasting window shifts your body to using body fat for fuel | When you avoid food for long periods of time you will probably eat fewer calories |
| Intermittent fasting (5:2 or alternate-day fasting) diets | During extended fasting, your body goes through even longer periods of burning body fat | When you avoid eating for entire days at a time, you will almost definitely eat fewer calories |
| Paleo diet | Only eating foods available to our cavemen ancestors is a surefire path to optimal health and weight | Prioritizing nutritious foods and avoiding high-calorie, highly processed foods will probably cause you to eat fewer calories |
| Almost every new fad diet you will ever see | Some sales pitch about how this works better than all other weight loss diets and you should definitely buy it | Whether they mention it or not, they are engineering different ways that encourage you to reduce your calorie intake |

## The Best Diet for You Does Not Need a Name

I feel the need to point out something that, in an ideal world, would be super-duper obvious, but unfortunately isn't as super-duper obvious as it should be. The nutritional approach you choose to follow doesn't actually need to have a name at all. If anything, I think this is a surprisingly underrated strategy. Let me paint you a picture to explain why.

The New Year rolls around and, inevitably, a whole wave of people decide they want to improve their health, and maybe lose a few pounds. Let's call one of those people Resolution Riley. Resolution Riley isn't sure what they should do, so they hop online and look for weight loss books available at their favorite online bookstore. What are they greeted with? A vast selection of different options, including all the ones we have discussed so far, plus some other lesser-known diet plans. A lot of them have catchy taglines like "the secret revolutionary way to get a six-pack with less time and effort than ever" or some sleazy sales shit like that. Resolution Riley isn't sure which one they should pick, but after clicking around for a bit they eventually opt for whichever one did the best marketing job and persuaded Riley that it contained the mystery recipe that they needed.

See, Riley was looking to handpick the diet that sounded most appealing to them—whichever diet looked the shiniest next to all the others, like choosing a diamond out of the rough. But you have done something different. You have read this chapter, which has laid out the whole menu of options next to each other. There have been no sales pitches or biased information to twist your arm, just a simplified summary of research so you know some pros and cons of each. I have done this for two main reasons. First, so you could pick a diet plan that works best for you. If you have read any of these sections and thought "Yes, that sounds right up my alley, I want to give that one a crack," then awesome, you have made your own informed decision, which is already a couple of steps above what Riley did. But, perhaps more importantly, by understanding how all popular weight loss diets work, you actually have the freedom to choose to do absolutely none of them at all.

You don't have to be one of those people who join the hardcore low-carb diet club or someone who goes around telling everyone they do intermittent fasting like it deserves a badge of honor. You don't need to follow a super strict Mediterranean or Paleo diet like your life depends on it. A lot of people join diet tribes, like they want to be part of a club where their favorite diet becomes their whole identity.

You could just pick and choose elements of different nutritional approaches that work for you without forcing yourself to follow any of these diets to the letter. If your goal is to lose body fat, you could reduce your portion sizes and actually keep everything you eat exactly the same. You could eat a bit more protein. You could swap some of the carbs you eat for more fruits and vegetables. You could reduce your intake of added oils by opting not to eat as much deep-fried food. You could reduce your alcohol intake and any snacks that you only eat out of boredom when you are in the office. You could just pick and choose individual behaviors and habits that are most effortless to you. One very well-known weight loss study didn't put all their participants on one specific brand fad diet, they just aimed for a 25 percent reduction in calorie intake and, alongside controlling portion sizes, they implemented certain strategies to make it easier to stick to.[102] These included prioritizing foods high in protein and fiber and favoring lower-calorie foods. Participants who followed this diet lost weight and improved several health markers without any significant adverse psychological effects.[103,104]

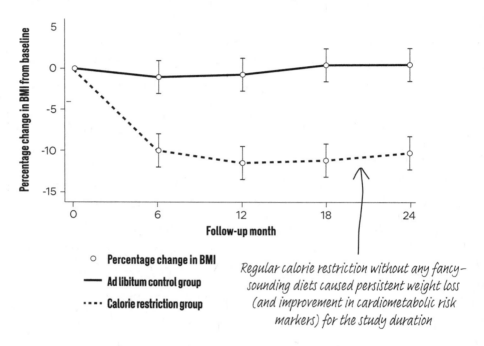

**Change in Body Mass Index (BMI) for the Ad Libitum Control Group and Calorie Restriction Group[105]**

Regular calorie restriction without any fancy-sounding diets caused persistent weight loss (and improvement in cardiometabolic risk markers) for the study duration

My hope is that, rather than blindly following one diet because it has great marketing or one that sounds appealing, you can actually handpick the specific elements of that diet that work best for you and disregard the elements that don't. In Chapter 5 we will discuss individual tips that overlap with some of these diets, plus some other healthy habits that don't, allowing you to create your own fully customized plan. First, though, I think it's important to do a self-audit so we know where you are now relative to where you would like to be.

# 4

# The Self-Audit

Imagine you want to hire me as your personal trainer. You slide into my email inbox and ask if I can coach you, so we work out a time and date for us to meet. You see me for the first time and we handshake or hug to greet (your choice, I am flexible). How would you feel if I handed you a new training program right away? Would you be taken aback, or would you just think I was being efficient? I know this might sound surprising, but I never *ever* go straight into training someone.

Say I asked you to do "15 reps of push-ups" as your first exercise. How do I know if that is appropriate for you? Some of you might not even be close to attempting a full push-up from the floor, while others might be push-up wizards who could easily bash out one hundred without breaking a sweat. Some of you might love push-ups and are happy I put them in your program, yet some of you might have pre-existing injuries that make doing push-ups a really bad idea. Are you starting to see the magnitude of the problem? This is precisely why I always like to know at least your rough training history before deciding anything. I want to see what your abilities are, what exercises you do and don't do, what your routine is like and various other things that give me a decent idea of where your program should start.

If something as simple as your workout routine should be customized to suit your goals, abilities and preferences, imagine how terrible it could be to give exactly the same nutritional advice to millions of people at once.

Chapters 5 and 6 set out the established habits and skills that can help you lose fat and keep it off. This chapter, with the self-audit questionnaires, is designed to mimic exactly what good professionals would do with you during an in-person appointment, finding solutions that are perfectly customized to you. So how does a self-audit work? The first step is establishing where you are now relative to where you would like to be, as it then allows us to understand what is standing in the way and gives us a much better chance of getting around it.

If you were a business management consultant and you walked into a struggling company with the goal of turning that around into something successful, what would you do? Would you just walk in, tell the staff to work harder and then leave? Of course not—that would be useless and probably patronizing advice because, for all you know, many of them are working hard already. Would you just tell them to earn more money and spend less money? No, that would also be shit guidance, because you haven't given them any kind of roadmap of how to achieve that. One of your first tasks would be to actually analyze the business and see where it needs improving so you can strategize how to help. If you've ever been blindly thrown a diet and exercise plan without someone taking the time to find out why you might be struggling in the first place, it wouldn't be surprising if that plan wasn't a magic solution after all. Have any diet books ever asked you to pause and think about reasons you might be finding it hard? Have any personal trainers ever told you to work harder but never asked what you are finding difficult and why? Well, fuck them for not bothering to take the time to understand you, and let's see if we can fix that.

As you already know from Chapter 2 where we discussed barriers and facilitators, there are a metric shit-ton of reasons why you might find it difficult to stick with nutrition and lifestyle changes, and these might be unique to you. The first thing we need to do is establish what they are. So, get comfortable, and I am going to pretend you are a real-life client. I will talk you through some of the questions I would ask if we were face-to-face. Needless to say, this is not intended to replace in-person advice from a relevant professional—like speaking to a registered dietitian for a personalized nutrition plan; it is just to plant some seeds for you to think about and hopefully they will grow into some useful lessons that can guide you on your path.

## Your Exercise and Dieting History

Diving into your history not only helps us find out what level you are at, but also tells us what you have tried in the past—for example, if there is anything you really enjoyed, or if there is anything you absolutely detested with every fiber of your being. As I have already mentioned, nearly half of adults have tried to lose weight recently,[1] so chances are most, if not all, of you reading this book have tried a few different diets before. Now, filling in whopping questionnaires is admittedly about as fun as watching paint dry, and I don't want to inflict that pain on you, so I have compiled a short list of questions that are adapted from the Weight and Lifestyle Inventory (WALI) questionnaire and the Emotional Eater Questionnaire (EEQ), which were both developed by respected professors and obesity researchers,[2,3] and the International Physical Activity Questionnaire (IPAQ), which was developed by an international consensus group.[4]

When you fill in questionnaires relating to physical activity, they often aren't brilliantly accurate for reflecting how much activity you actually did.[5] There are many reasons for this, a key one being that, when we recall things from memory, we have a tendency to round up. For example, even though it's part of my job, I don't actually know how many minutes I exercised this week. I could guess, but it's highly possible I won't be quite right. This is also the same with questionnaires asking you about what you eat. It is extraordinarily difficult to fully trust the answers people give you.[6] Firstly, if I asked you to write down every single meal and snack you ate this week, I reckon 99 percent of you would forget at least one thing. Personally, I need to think hard to remember what I ate for dinner five days ago, let alone every single snack I have nibbled on. Secondly, even if you did remember everything you ate, it is normal to have to guess at portion sizes. Was that one serving or two that you ate? Was that a full serving of vegetables or just half? Was that 50g (1¾oz) of chocolate you ate after dinner or 100g (3½oz)? Statistically speaking, the likelihood people can record their calorie intake to any high degree of accuracy hovers only a teeny bit above zero, as most people have a tendency to significantly underreport what they eat.[7] Imagine what happens when you ask people how many servings of several different food groups they eat in an average week and then consider that this might be totally different to what it was six months ago. Long story short, please consider the physical activity and dietary questions as ballpark estimates. They are not going to be perfectly precise, but something doesn't have to be precise to still be useful. If anything, trying to be too precise can come with a level of obsession that is worth steering clear of, which we will discuss in Chapter 7 when we talk about calorie counting.

If you're reading the print version of this book, feel free to scribble in it if you fancy. If you're reading the digital ebook version, grab a piece of paper or open a notes app to jot down your answers. Alternatively, if you are listening to the audiobook, you can look at the accompanying PDF file. Of course, if you just can't be bothered to write anything down, at least pause for a moment to consider your answers.

## Weight history and goals

1. To help us establish your dieting history, what nutrition and lifestyle strategies have you followed that have resulted in a weight loss of 4.5kg (10lb) or more? (By this I mean intentional dieting only, so you don't need to include the time you got food poisoning and spent a week emptying the entire contents of your digestive system or anything like that.)

2. In the past year, how many times have you embarked on an intentional weight loss program? This includes diets of any duration, whether you followed something for several months or just tried it for a couple of days.

3. Have you ever experienced any significant negative side effects from trying to lose weight? These can be physical or emotional; whatever you remember. If yes, what were your symptoms?

4. Do you currently have a weight or fat loss goal? If so, how much would you like to lose?

5. When did you last weigh your target weight and how long did you maintain it?

### Lifestyle

1. Do you currently smoke? If so, how many cigarettes per day? Feel free to say how many you smoke per month if you don't smoke daily.

2. If you have ever smoked and then stopped, did you notice any weight gain? If so, how much, roughly?

3. Do you currently drink alcohol? If so, how many drinks do you have per week? If you drink less frequently, how many do you have per month?

4. Do you take any other recreational drugs? No judgment. As these can obviously affect your health, it can be a useful thing to know when designing your plan.

### Eating habits

1. Do you find that social factors affect your health and weight, such as eating with family and friends or when socializing, celebrating or at business events?

2. Do you eat because you love the taste of food?

3. Do you crave specific foods?

4. Do you ever overeat at breakfast, lunch or dinner? Note if it is one meal in particular.

5. Do you snack a lot between meals or after dinner?

6. Do you feel like weighing scales hold a power over you and can affect your mood?

7. Do emotions affect when you eat, such as when you are stressed, angry, bored, sad, depressed, anxious or lonely?

8. Do you feel guilty if you eat "forbidden" foods?

9. Does being tired affect your ability to have control over your diet?

10. If you think you've eaten too much while on a diet, do you tend to give up, feel like you've lost control and eat more?

11. How many times do you eat per week? Add up your breakfasts, lunches, dinners and snacks.

12. What does your diet look like on a typical weekday?

13. What does your diet look like on a typical weekend?

### Physical activity

During a typical week:

1. How many minutes of vigorous activity do you do? This can include things like running, fast cycling and heavy lifting.

2. How many minutes of moderate intensity activity do you do? Only include things you do for more than ten minutes at a time, like cycling at a regular pace, carrying light loads or playing doubles tennis.

3. How many minutes do you spend walking?

4. How many minutes do you spend sitting?

5. Do you enjoy any of the following forms of exercise? Walking outside, walking on the treadmill, jogging, running, cycling outside, cycling inside, group aerobics classes, racket sports, swimming, basketball, golf, dancing, weight lifting? Others? Please describe.

These questionnaires won't cover every aspect of your health and lifestyle. The aim is to provide you with sample questions that will help you understand the key areas without having to spend a load of time filling in the full versions.

First, they allow us (because you and I are a team now, obviously) to assess where you are starting from nutrition- and exercise-wise. This then lays the groundwork for goal-setting and habit change that is *actually* personalized, rather than some shitty identical cookie-cutter copy-and-paste program that inevitably isn't suitable for most people.

Second, I wanted to include some sample questions from an emotional eating questionnaire to get you thinking about *why* you might struggle to change your food intake. Some people think dieting is easy-peasy, and maybe it is for them. But, as we will discuss in Chapter 6 on how to support healthy habits, many others find it extremely difficult because their appetite, food cravings and ability to manage what they eat can be influenced by a fuckload of different behind-the-scenes factors. For example, you might be someone who resorts to "comfort eating" in response to emotional stress. If you feel stressed a lot, it's possible that you will not only eat more food, but also gravitate toward delicious high-calorie treats specifically.[8] This is a simple example of why emotional eating is often linked with weight gain,[9] but it also shows why focusing on addressing emotional triggers may be important in increasing your likelihood of weight loss success. For example, one research study concluded that the odds of weight loss success after 12 months were 1.7 times higher for participants who decreased their emotional eating than those whose emotional eating increased, causing the researchers to claim "A reduction in emotional eating may be critical to weight loss success."[10] Another study reported that half of people who dieted and regained weight attributed that yo-yo regain to at least one emotional reason.[11]

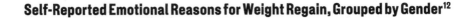

## Self-Reported Emotional Reasons for Weight Regain, Grouped by Gender[12]

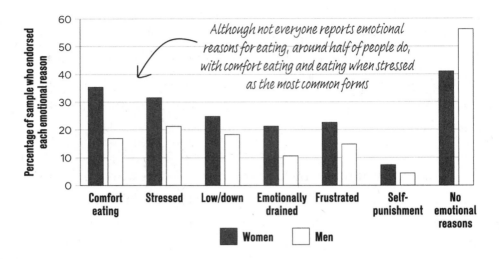

*Although not everyone reports emotional reasons for eating, around half of people do, with comfort eating and eating when stressed as the most common forms*

## Why Do Your Goals Actually Motivate You?

When I was a teenager, I remember setting myself an exercise goal to lift a certain weight in the gym (on bench press obviously, because teenage gym bros always love training their chest, and I was no exception). My whole exercise experience immediately became more fun. I was excited to go to the gym, and I felt happier every time I tracked a tiny improvement on my journey to that goal. I wasn't just going to the gym, I was going to the gym with a purpose.

Have you ever had a target that was so similarly exciting that you really knuckled down and worked your arse off to try to achieve it? Setting goals for yourself can be an amazingly powerful tool. But it can also be a fucking terrible tool when used improperly, and it's important to understand some pros and cons.

Having weight loss targets is often linked to better results,[13] but it is also extraordinarily common for people to set unrealistic goals for themselves.[14,15] For example, in one research study, a group of women aimed at numbers that were so overly ambitious, nearly half of them failed to even hit their "disappointed" weight loss targets, let alone their "reasonable," "happy" or "dream" weight loss goals.[16] This does not mean that if you are too ambitious you will automatically be shooting yourself in the foot,[17] but it is worth being aware of.

### Participant Expectations[18]

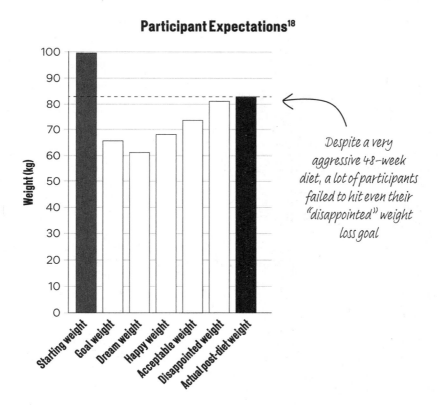

Despite a very aggressive 48-week diet, a lot of participants failed to hit even their "disappointed" weight loss goal

Although the most common questions around weight loss are things like, "How much weight do you want to lose?," "What size clothing would you like to wear?," "When would you like to achieve this by?" and "When did you last weigh this amount?," I would like to ask a different question. I would like to ask you *why* you have the goal (or goals) that you do, and I actually want to ask it five times. This is not an interrogation technique. It's just an empathetic attempt to understand what really motivates you to have the goal that you do. The "five whys" method is a simple tool to help identify the real root of a problem,[19] but it can also be used to find the underlying reasons you have the ambitions that you do. Let me give you an example of why I like to use it.

### The "five whys" method

Let's say Fictitious Frankie comes to me and says, "Ben, I really want to lose some weight."

"OK, **why** would you like to lose weight?"

"I want to feel healthier."

"**Why** do you want to feel healthier?"

"Well, I notice I get out of breath quickly."

"**Why** does that matter to you?"

"I think I would feel better if my fitness improved."

"**Why** is that?"

"Well, I get embarrassed when I am working out."

"**Why** does that matter?"

"Because it stops me from going to the gym because I am worried people are judging me."

Over the years, many clients have approached me with a goal, but their underlying motivation is actually a little bit different once you peel back the layers of the metaphorical onion. Sometimes a guy says he wants to build muscle, but his real motivation is to stop feeling self-conscious when he takes off his top. Sometimes people tell me they want to lose weight, but their deeper motivation is not about seeing a lower number on the scales, it's that they think losing weight might make them feel fitter and healthier, or help them live longer, or maybe even make them more attractive to other people or jazz up their sex life. So, take a moment to think about your goals. What made you look at this book and think, "Yes, I think I need that in my life," and then ask yourself why those goals matter to you. You might be surprised by what your final answer is after a little bit of self-reflection.

Let's flip the roles, and I will give you a brutally honest personal insight into my own goal motivations. I started working out when I was about 15 or 16 years old, just doing random workouts like sit-ups and push-ups in my bedroom because I wanted to grow some muscle. Looking back, I think I was maybe a little bit insecure as I wasn't exactly the biggest hit with the girls at my school. As I started getting more muscular, I noticed that more people complimented me on the way that I looked, which fueled me to keep going. To begin with, I liked that I could see my body changing, but, over time, the extrinsic motivations dissipated (which is probably a good thing). After a few years, I noticed my progress slowed down a lot (which tends to happen when you have been lifting weights for a long time and don't secretly use performance-enhancing drugs), but my motivation to exercise was firmly ingrained. Nowadays, I train because I love the feeling of getting stronger and fitter. That is particularly important to me because I have a chronic disease that terrifies me, so I try my best to stay healthy as I get older. I have been through periods of my life when my disease flare-ups were so painful I struggled to get out of bed, let alone work out. This gave me an extra motivation to hold on to fitness, strength and muscle mass as much as possible to try to give myself an extra fighting chance if that ever happens to me again.

My original goal as a teenager to get more muscular has drifted a bit, but exercise has become a habitual thing that I enjoy, and that fundamental motivation might not only be important for exercise consistency (yay),[20] but also for having better body image (double yay),[21] which is why exercising exclusively to change the way you look probably isn't a super smart idea. If you know what fuels your motivational fire, it can help you strategize the best ways of keeping it burning bright. Personally, I love seeing progress by numbers. Getting a little bit stronger or being able to jog a little bit faster or for a little bit longer are things that excite me because I love the feeling of making measurable progress. If you challenged me to lift 5kg (11lb) more on an exercise within 30 days, that would increase my enjoyment far more than exercising just for the sake of it, even if the workout plan looked identical on paper.

## Where Do You Want to Go and What Will It Cost?

A client came to me once and told me they wanted to look like the guy on the front cover of a men's fitness magazine. I told him that this was very possible, and I outlined the type of intense training routine that it would require. Leading up to photoshoots, a lot of fitness models train twice per day; some take performance-enhancing drugs, follow very restrictive diets and even sacrifice their own health to achieve a temporarily low level of body fat just for photoshoot purposes. I was not trying to dissuade my client from that goal; I simply wanted to tell him about the costs in an unbiased fashion and let him make his own decisions. Once I had done this, he basically said, "Fuck that, it sounds miserable." Instead, we talked about what was realistic for him to achieve without him having to do the extreme stuff that professional fitness models frequently resort to.

In this chapter, we are doing the book equivalent of you sitting with me and having a chat about your goals. Hopefully, you have an idea of where you are now, and not only what you want, but also why you want it. One remaining thing I like to ask my new clients is about the price they are willing to pay to achieve that goal. If someone told you they wanted to become a multimillionaire CEO, but said they didn't want to work long hours or be stressed a lot of the time, you would probably advise them to recalibrate their expectations and pick a goal more suited to them. If they wanted to work hard, it's totally possible they could climb the career ladder, but if they want a stress-free job, chances are the CEO of a mega corporation isn't a role that would fill their happiness bucket. Ideally, we want goals that will actually enrich our lives rather than accidentally sabotaging them.

The idea here is to pair the goals you want to achieve with the habits coming in Chapter 5 that you are happy to embark on. Obviously, there will be some discrepancies between your future goals and your current behaviors (because if you were already doing everything necessary, you probably wouldn't be reading this book in the first place). This is a concept commonly used within something called motivational interviewing, which is sometimes used alongside weight loss treatments,[22,23,24,25] the goal of which is to help facilitate and promote the likelihood of successful behavior change by increasing your own levels of self-efficacy and intrinsic motivation. This sounds nerdy, but it is actually quite straightforward. When I doubt my own ability to achieve something, talking to my wife about what I am struggling with often makes me feel like I can actually do it, which then makes me far more inclined to take action toward my goal. On the flip side, there might be people in your life who hold you back or make you doubt yourself, which makes you less confident that you can accomplish the thing you have in your head. Breaking big, insurmountable-feeling tasks into more manageable behaviors is a little bit like working out how to scale the metaphorical mountain rather than just standing at the bottom and telling yourself that you cannot climb it.

To finish this self-audit chapter, I invite you to spend a few minutes completing the questions on pages 113 and 114. Once again, feel free to scribble your answers in this book or use a notepad or digital notes app if you are reading the ebook or listening to the audiobook.

It is commonly claimed that writing down your goals increases the likelihood of you achieving them, and you might see suspiciously specific percentages thrown out there like "Writing down your goals increases your chance of hitting them by 42 percent," and I think that's a bit silly. After all, surely it depends on a bazillion different factors, including what your actual goal is. If one hundred of you wrote down that you wanted to walk one mile per day and one hundred of you said you wanted to be the next president of the United States, I suspect the percentage success rate would differ a smidge. If I wrote down that my goal was to be the first man who unicycles on the moon, I am not super sure it would be more likely to come to fruition. That being said, there are some examples in research literature where people who set any goal type appeared to have improved academic performance compared to people who didn't, on average, and this included writing them down.[26,27]

Although skeptical, when I first heard this advice over ten years ago, I wrote down my goals on a small piece of paper and stuck it to the wall above my kitchen sink. The theory is, seeing your goals written down can increase your sense of enthusiasm and focus your attention toward them and away from goal-irrelevant activities.[28] For example, if you write a to-do list each morning, it becomes crystal clear what you need to focus on for the day in priority order, which may also have the additional effect of you being able to tune out less-important tasks. I saw my list of goals every single day, and it served as a continual reminder of what I wanted to achieve to make that year a great year. For me personally, it had a far more positive impact on my motivation, my overall well-being and my accomplishments than my cynical brain originally suspected. This is why goal-setting is often encouraged across a wide range of endeavors,[29] but also specifically used for healthy behavior change interventions, including weight loss.[30]

Given that you spent some of your hard-earned pennies on this book, I figure it's worth taking a few minutes to complete an easy task, especially if it might help you gain clarity on what you want to achieve, why you want to achieve it and what you think you might need to do to get there. If it helps increase your chances of success then it will have been a few minutes that were extremely well spent.

### Setting health goals

What goals are important to you? Bonus points if they are specific and measurable.

*For example, "get faster at jogging" is vague, but "be able to jog one mile in under eight minutes by December 31" is specific.*

Why are these goals important to you? Use the five whys process we discussed earlier to think about the deeper reasons why these goals motivate you.

### Current habit analysis

What healthy habits are you already doing that positively impact your life? Use the self-audit questions to help you answer this.

In which areas do you see room for improvement? Consider any discrepancies between your current behaviors and future goals.

Are there any obstacles you need to overcome? Look back at the subsection on barriers and facilitators (see page 43).

The self-audit in this chapter has helped you determine your starting point. In the next chapter, I'll set out 13 established healthy habits you can use as tools to help you reach your desired destination of improving your health, losing body fat and keeping it off.

# 5

# Choosing Your Fat Loss Habits

A lot of weight loss books are marketed by saying they have some kind of revolutionary, never-heard-of-before diet plan you all need to follow to get the best results and, as you hopefully now realize from Chapter 3, where we discussed different diets, that is absolute horse shit. If there really was one magic diet that definitely solved all of your problems, then the scientists who discovered it would be telling you all for free. I would be making countless free videos on social media about those research studies, doing my best to shout about it from the rooftops.

The truth is, the shit that works best is actually very simple and it is in front of our eyes already: reducing your calorie intake, reducing your intake of ultra-processed foods that are high in added sugars, added fats and calories, exercising more, eating more fruits and vegetables, and eating more protein. While these methods don't sound very exciting, they fucking work. The real problem we need to solve is how we actually take this basic-sounding information and make sure you can put it into action, consistently. For example, we know that exercise is good. I imagine every adult on the planet already knows it is great for our health, right? Even though we all universally know this, do you know how many people *actually* perform the recommended target for aerobic and resistance training combined? One research study comprised data of over 3 million participants spanning 32 countries and concluded it's in the region of an abysmal 17 percent.[1] Another study looked at global trends of physical activity across 168 different countries and found that, between 2001 and 2016, there was no significant uptick in what percentage of adults performed enough exercise. In 2013 the member states of the WHO set a target to reduce the relative prevalence of physical inactivity by just 10 percent by 2025, yet, as a global population, we failed to get on track to hit even this modest goal.[2] There is a vast chasm between what we know we need to do to improve our health and our ability to actually put that shit into action. This is where the idea of habits comes in.

No one pretends the individual habits in this chapter are revolutionary. None of them are brand-new information to anyone who reads a lot of fat loss research literature. These are 13 fundamental habits that often get overlooked in an industry full of people saying they have a shiny cutting-edge solution for your needs. Nobody actually has a magic key that unpicks the seemingly impossible lock. The real key is learning how to implement the behaviors we already know work, and managing to do so for the rest of our lives. That's the secret bit most diet books never even talk about.

## Why Habits?

I think willpower is overrated. Too many people talk about it like it's the key to unlocking a secret world of health benefits. "If only you had more willpower to go to the gym"; "If only you had more willpower to eat less chocolate"; blah, blah, blah. As we have discussed previously, people don't gain weight simply because they have some kind of willpower deficiency.[3] If your body fat percentage is higher than mine, this doesn't automatically mean you are lazier than I am. Perhaps I have better genetics. Perhaps I just find it easier to follow certain behaviors. Willpower can play a role, obviously, but telling people that they "just need more willpower" is about as useful as a chocolate teapot. It just doesn't fucking work.[4]

What actually is willpower? Although many people talk about it, its strict definition is sometimes argued. One research paper offers this explanation: "Willpower is the process of overcoming a seemingly superior, currently available smaller, sooner reward to get a larger, later alternative."[5] In the 1960s, a very simple series of studies became one of the most famous psychological experiments ever, now known as the "marshmallow test." In an attempt to measure children's ability to delay gratification, preschoolers were offered one little treat now, or they could wait to eat two treats later.[6] In theory, if they could resist the urge to eat one mini marshmallow knowing they could eat two mini marshmallows instead, this would demonstrate self-control in the face of temptation. This is an example of exerting willpower. Doing it in the short term can be hard, so expecting to do it repeatedly to execute a difficult action every single day for the rest of your life is always going to be an uphill battle. If you were really hungry and I put your favorite snack in front of you, it would take a lot of willpower for you to resist that snack. Or if you were exhausted from a long day at work, and needed to drag yourself off the couch so you could go to the gym, that would also take willpower. Think of it like self-control. You are overriding your natural temptations because you want to reach your goals. But constantly exerting willpower to fight your urges is about as fun as rubbing lemon juice in your eyes. So, maybe a better question is: What other strategies can you use rather than simply relying on willpower for the rest of your life?[7]

What if you became so consistently good at doing something that it became a subconscious habit, and it no longer required you to exert huge amounts of willpower to do it? Going to the gym when you hate going to the gym requires a lot of your willpower. But what if, over a period of time, you began to love going to the gym? Well, it would require less willpower for you to go, because you wouldn't be fighting your natural temptation to avoid it, right? The goal is: how can we make habits feel effortless for you, so you have a better chance of maintaining them in the long run?

In 1890, William James wrote this in a book called *The Principles of Psychology*: "We must make automatic and habitual, as early as possible, as many useful actions as we can...The more of the details of our daily life we can hand over to the effortless custody of automatism, the more our higher powers of mind will be set free for their own proper work."[8]

Achieving better outcomes does not always mean you exerted more willpower. It often just means you adopted better systems that actually decreased your need for willpower in the first place. If you can take the most fundamental and beneficial behaviors and turn them into habits that become second nature, you won't need to buy another overhyped diet plan again.

Before we go into healthy habits in more detail, it is also important to understand that behavior change can also include breaking so-called bad habits. Someone going from sedentary to exercising for the first time is adopting a new, health-promoting habit, but they may also want to break lingering habits like watching a lot of television. This is not where we are going to spend the majority of this chapter, because the actual research on breaking bad habits in the context of health and weight management is extremely slim. However, here are some good things to understand.

In research literature, habits are often more like automatic responses to situations and contextual cues that largely happen outside of your conscious awareness.[9] For example, if you grab snacks every time you sit down to watch a movie, watching a movie has become the cue for you to eat snacks, and chances are you do this without even really thinking about it.

So, what are some different strategies to break habits that no longer serve you? Here are some simple examples:[10]

- Habit discontinuation: Avoid the cues in the first place. Remove yourself from the environment that cues the unwanted habit. If you want to stop gambling, not setting foot in a casino makes sense. In the context of nutrition, if you don't like that you stop by the same cake shop every time you walk past it on the way to work, walking a different route can remove that cue of you seeing the cake shop.

- Habit inhibition: Rather than avoiding the situation altogether, you can monitor something and aim to improve on it over time, like students who monitor how much they procrastinate by watching the television and gradually inhibit that behavior, rather than throwing their TV out of the window (this is one reason the self-audit chapter is so important, and we will talk about monitoring in the next chapter).

- Habit substitution: Displace a previous reaction to a cue with a new one. If you always finish dinner and immediately turn to dessert, eating dinner is essentially reinforced as the cue for your sweet tooth. Rather than expecting to stop eating dessert altogether (discontinuation), or slowly eating less dessert because you are aware of it (inhibition), you can substitute it by eating a preferred food. For example, instead of eating a snack high in added sugars after my lunch, I swapped it for a couple of pieces of fruit. Years later, as soon as I finish eating lunch, my brain still automatically wants to grab a piece of fruit. This is a habit that took willpower at the beginning, but, over time, repeating this new habit substitution took less and less effort to the point that it became automatic.

## A Decision Tree to Aid Selection of Habit Change Strategies[11]

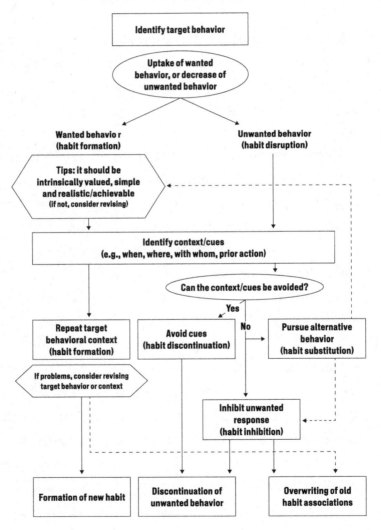

Now that you have the express summary of how to break or decrease bad habits, let's move on to the main topic, which has a lot more research literature to discuss: the beneficial behaviors that I would love for you to adopt consistently enough for them to become habitual.

### How to build a healthy habit

To build a framework for implementing a healthy habit, start with deciding on a goal—use the goal-setting questions in the previous chapter. From here, one research paper suggested choosing a simple action, and picking a time and place to do this action daily. Be consistent and it will become easier over time: "You might start noticing yourself doing it automatically without having to think about it. It might take as little as ten weeks for some, while others will progress faster or slower depending on their personal circumstances."[12]

For example, rather than saying, "I want to earn more money," which is a vague outcome goal, you can focus on the individual behaviors that will help you achieve that: checking your savings and expenses regularly to monitor cash flow, removing any unnecessary expenses that you realize are costing too much, learning a new side hustle if your job doesn't have any options for career progression, and so on. As a weight loss example, if you have a goal to lose weight and improve your health, one of the individual behaviors that help support that might be eating more fruits and vegetables. A simple action that includes the time and place might be to put a piece of fruit on your desk each morning and eat this after lunch every day. If you do this consistently, it will eventually start becoming a subconscious habit that requires less cognitive effort and it will feel more instinctive. A personal example is when I first started taking Korean lessons so I could talk to my wife's family more easily; I used to practice for just 15 minutes a day. It wasn't a lot, but it was way easier than trying to squeeze hour-long classes into my work schedule. I did it on my phone when I first got into bed and, over time, that became habitual for me. Now it's become an effortless activity I do every day, often for much longer periods of time. It takes me far less mental energy to complete a higher volume of work than it did when I started, which is a testament to ingraining behaviors into your subconscious routine. A lot of people exercise first thing in the morning after their coffee and before they go to work, not because they have sky-high levels of willpower throughout their life, but simply because they have embedded this into their daily routine so deeply that it doesn't hurt like it used to. Ask anyone who has been going to the gym for decades why they keep going, and chances are they are going to tell you that it's just an automatic part of their routine. Set your own goal and action plan below.

My goal...

My plan...

Some research studies have tested this kind of super-simple "habit formation" advice to see if it could help promote weight loss.[13,14] Rather than putting people on an extreme and restrictive diet like most weight loss advice tends to default to, you can give them a basic leaflet with ten healthy habits. The goal is simple: try to get better at consistently slotting those habits into your routine, like the framework we've just discussed. Here were the habits they followed:

1. Eat five servings of fruits and vegetables daily.
2. Don't stack food high on your plate.
3. Check food labels to decrease your intake of foods high in added sugars and added fats.
4. If you love snacks, swap your less nutritious ones for more nutritious ones like fruit and yogurt instead of candy and chocolate.
5. Reduce your alcohol and sugary soda intake in favor of water or other lower-calorie drinks.
6. Do not eat while distracted, like when watching TV.
7. Where possible, favor lower fat foods like leaner cuts of meat over fattier cuts of meat.
8. Keep your regular meal routine, regardless of what that currently is.
9. Walk 10,000 steps daily.
10. If you spend a lot of time sitting, interrupt each hour of sitting time with 10 minutes on your feet.

You might notice that they weren't told to count every calorie they ate. They weren't told which foods they needed to avoid like the plague. They weren't told to do intermittent fasting or whatever fad diet was trending at the time. They weren't even told to do anything that aggressive at all. They were just told to follow ten basic habits, and these were enough to start promoting mild weight loss; all as a result of giving people a leaflet with simple, easy-to-follow instructions. This is the concept behind habit-based weight loss interventions.[15,16]

Some of you might look at the list of habits above and think, "Holy shit, that sounds perfect for me." Depending on your goals, where you are now and where you want to be, these might be ten great habits you want to follow with the perfect cost-to-benefit ratio for you. But some of you might think, "Nah, I want something different" or "A few of those don't really grab my attention," so let's make this more interactive. After all, I want this book you spent your hard-earned pennies on to be a lot more thorough and personalized than an identical leaflet given to dozens of people, like they did in the research study.

Let's pretend you and I decide to go on holiday. I am letting you take the lead because I want you to be in charge of where you go and my job is just to help you get there. You have picked somewhere exciting (which is why the previous goal-setting chapter was so important), either a new adventure or a place you've been dying to revisit. The destination looks great, so what would be the first step in making this trip a reality? Now is the time to decide the best way of getting there.

You might be the type of person who is desperate to arrive as fast as possible and you couldn't give a shit how uncomfortable the journey might be. You are happy to leave now and travel through the night if that's what it takes because you just care about getting there. Some of you would prefer to take things slower, because rushing seems unnecessarily stressful and that doesn't tickle your proverbial pickle. You might be the kind of person who wants to plan the journey at a more sociable time of the day, via a more comfortable method of transport. It might take a little longer, but it's more enjoyable for you. There is no right or wrong here, just your own personal preference.

You're in charge of your own journey. I can advise, but ultimately you should do what is best for you. The most important thing to understand is that a lot of people are so desperate to get from A to B that they do it via any means necessary, and sometimes they find out the journey sucks a lot more than they thought it would. Sometimes it sucks so much that they don't get from A to B at all. They get halfway along the route, realize that the method of transport they picked is unbearable and decide to just bugger off back home instead.

In this chapter, I am going to give you a list of 13 possible behaviors and explain their rationale. Think of these like a menu. You can ignore anything that looks too expensive for you or not to your taste and pick the things that sound appealing and feel achievable. Hopefully, if you try a few different options, you might find the big winner, or two, you want to keep using. Your goal is to select behaviors to do more or less of and get consistent enough at them that they take less effort than they used to. If you can ingrain healthy habits so deeply that they become second nature to you, *that* is the real key to lifelong change.

## The Habits

Pick a handful of behaviors that 1) appeal to you personally, 2) are realistic for you to implement, and 3) are powerful enough to take you toward your goal if you implement them consistently. Of course, these can be combined with any of the dietary strategies we discussed in Chapter 3, if that is right for you and your goals. You don't need to overexert yourself by trying to go from zero to hero straightaway. The goal is to go from square one, to square two, to square three, and so on. Over time, as you practice your habits more and more, they should start becoming second nature and require less conscious effort to stick to them, at which point you can always add another habit if you want.

## Habit 1: Prioritize nutritious lower-energy-density foods

As we briefly mentioned in Chapter 3, "energy density" just means the number of calories per gram of food. It is very important to understand this concept before discussing the following habits. Let me use an extreme example to explain energy density: 100g (or 3.5oz) of cucumber contains fewer than 20 calories, but the same 100g of the delicious cookies I have in my cupboard right now (about half a pack) contains nearly 500 calories. If you put those 500 calories' worth of cookies into a bowl, it would look like a very reasonably sized snack. But, if you wanted to eat the same 500 calories from the cucumber, you would be eating somewhere in the region of a dozen whole cucumbers, which I think is fair to describe as an unreasonably large portion for any regular human. I could happily eat that half-pack of cookies and still want to keep going, but I have never ever sat down and thought to myself, "I just really fancy eating 12 whole cucumbers this evening."

These foods, from opposite ends of the spectrum, are useful examples to help you understand the concept of energy density. It sounds simple, but it actually underpins a lot of dietary advice, even though most plans never mention it explicitly.

- If a diet plan tells you to eat more fruits and vegetables, these are foods that have a low energy density, so they tend to be good for appetite regulation.
- If a diet plan tells you to avoid ultra-processed foods, this is because they tend to have a high energy density and are easy to eat in excess.
- If a diet plan tells you to limit added fats, like grilling food instead of frying, and not using a lot of oils and salad dressings, this lowers the energy density of those meals.

- If a diet plan tells you to trim the fat off meat or look for leaner cuts of red meat, this reduces the energy density of those meals.
- If a diet plan tells you to avoid sugary drinks in favor of water, it is because sugary drinks all have a much higher energy density than water, which contains zero calories.

Basically, there are a shitload of different ways to manipulate your diet that hinge on the underlying principle of reducing its overall energy density. Doing this can gently steer you toward eating fewer calories,[17] which can then help you to lose weight.[18]

Knowing this concept makes you smart, but knowing the best ways to implement it makes you even smarter. After all, I could say, "Every time you want a cookie, a doughnut or some chocolate, eat cucumber slices instead" and that would indeed reduce the energy density of your diet, but it would also rapidly reduce your will to live. After all, if you have a cookie-shaped hole in your heart, I doubt any amount of cucumber is ever going to fill it. So, I would like you to think about changes and swaps that are painless because the benefit always has to outweigh the cost.

For example, swapping your burger bun for a lettuce leaf is becoming quite a popular calorie-saving tip and I have even seen it on offer at some restaurants, but just seeing a burger wrapped in lettuce makes me feel sad, let alone being the one trying to eat it. It might appeal to some people, but that one doesn't seem like a painless swap to me. Using diced cauliflower as "rice" or very thinly sliced courgette (that's zucchini in America) as "spaghetti" has also taken off as a bit of a trend, and I actually see both of these sold in grocery stores—but again, I would rather just eat the real thing. If I am making a delicious curry at home, serving it over minced cauliflower instead of a nice mound of rice is a surefire way to ruin that dinner I have prepared. Trying to "save calories" sounds great and all, but not when it comes with a huge expense of enjoyment. Have you ever followed a diet plan and just found yourself feeling miserable with the food choices because you had to eat things you hated, or you were prohibited from eating foods you loved? How long did that diet last? You aren't likely to keep doing something if it's too painful, right?

Where possible, I also strongly prefer to focus on what you can do more of rather than what you need to do less of. Whatever you do, try not to think of a big, bright pink elephant. Definitely don't imagine what it looks like. Chances are, you haven't thought of a big, bright pink elephant at all recently because why would you? But, when I mention it, you have to think about it even if the goal is not to think about it. Anecdotally, many people find that when they are told to avoid certain foods during a diet, it almost feels like they think about them more and it becomes seemingly impossible to avoid them for long periods of time.

Some people say "absence makes the heart grow fonder," so if you love pizza and you have tried to avoid it when dieting only to feel like your cravings for pizza are higher than ever, maybe avoiding the pizza completely is not a smart strategy for you. This is an ongoing debate, but the idea is that the initial restriction can backfire and you can find yourself eating even more of it than you would regularly, and some of you may be more susceptible to this phenomenon than others.[19] I have lost count of the number of clients who have come to me and said something like, "I really love chocolate, but every time I cut it out, I can only do it for a couple of weeks before I find myself binge eating it," and it doesn't take a genius to know that binge eating is not the desired consequence of reducing your chocolate intake. Binge eating is a common predictor of eating more food and gaining weight,[20] so if you go through periods of restricting a food and then binge eating it, it can be a bit like taking two steps forward and then three steps back. A lot of diets revolve around food avoidance, restriction, deprivation and misery, so sometimes it can feel like a nice change to focus on the positive things you can add rather than constantly obsessing about negative things you need to avoid.

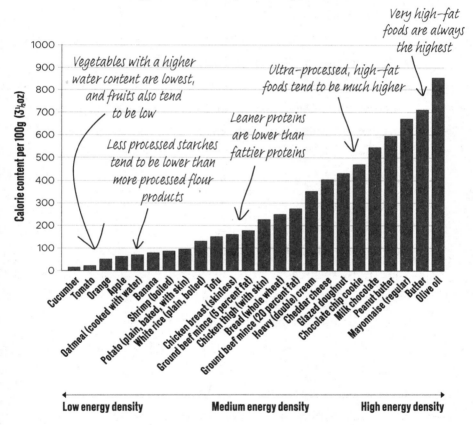

**Energy Density Examples of Popular Foods**

Very high-fat foods are always the highest

Vegetables with a higher water content are lowest, and fruits also tend to be low

Ultra-processed, high-fat foods tend to be much higher

Less processed starches tend to be lower than more processed flour products

Leaner proteins are lower than fattier proteins

Calorie content per 100g (3½oz)

Low energy density    Medium energy density    High energy density

Adopting any of the following strategies will help you develop habitual behaviors that prioritize low-energy-density foods:

- Reduce your intake of high-calorie ultra-processed foods, as reiterated by several of the different diet plans that we discussed in Chapter 3, in favor of more nutritious, less processed foods. I cannot overstate the importance of this, and if you can do it consistently it's quite possibly the most important habit that you can nail, which will improve your health and promote fat loss via a reduction in calorie intake.

- If reducing or eliminating these foods is something you have struggled with in the past, focus on prioritizing your preferred nutritious foods and let these naturally displace lesser preferred foods out of your diet. For example, many people eat most of their high-calorie foods in the evening as dessert, which is often because they are still hungry after dinner. Eating more of the (hopefully) nutritious foods you eat for dinner can make you less hungry for dessert, naturally displacing those high-calorie foods, which then take up less of your overall diet. Based on your self-audit in the previous chapter, you have probably identified areas you might want to change.

- You can also swap certain foods in favor of others at each meal. For example, less processed wholegrains like oatmeal are often better for appetite regulation than ultra-processed grains like sugary cereal, which are common at breakfast. Less processed rice and potato products are often better for appetite regulation and have a lower energy density than ultra-processed bread products and pizzas, which are common at dinner.

We will discuss other more specific strategies in the next three habits.

## Habit 2: Eat more fruits and vegetables

Take a wild guess at what percentage of adults don't eat enough fruits and vegetables? Maybe 50 percent? Perhaps even higher, like 70 percent? Actually, by some estimates, it's even higher. Using a big country like America as an example, nearly 90 percent of adults are falling short.[21] On average, only one in ten adults hits the recommended targets for fruits and vegetables, but this is especially pronounced when people have less money, because if you are really tight for cash and struggling to feed your family, you probably don't give a shit about buying an extra bag of kale. You just want to make sure your family is consuming enough food first, rather than trying to decorate that food with nearly zero-calorie green leafy vegetables.

Fruits and vegetables can contain an array of vitamins, minerals and bioactive compounds, plus fiber, and people who eat more of them not only tend to be healthier,[22] but they also tend to live longer.[23] Do you *need* to eat them to lose body fat? Absolutely not. Technically, you also don't need to exercise to lose body fat, but that doesn't stop it from being a great fucking idea. Fruits and vegetables are wonderful for health reasons and many diets only focus on trying to reduce the number on the scales, rather than giving two shits about your overall health and well-being.

On top of beneficial stuff like vitamins and minerals, fruits and vegetables have a low energy density because they tend to be very high in water, which is why tomatoes, cucumber and celery contain barely any calories. Due to their high water and low calorie content, telling people to eat more of them can inadvertently promote weight loss, even when you do not tell people how many calories to eat. For example, if you tell people to reduce their fat intake and eat more fruits and vegetables, they can lose weight even if you don't tell them to bother worrying about calories at all.[24]

Research has shown some very easy ways to do this. Let's pretend you have a plateful of food in front of you and it is roughly 50 percent protein and 50 percent carbohydrates, like beef and rice, or whatever is easy to imagine. If someone told you to eat a smaller portion of both, that already sounds miserable because who wants to eat a tiny child's portion of food? But instead, how about you keep the same size portion, but let a vegetable like broccoli displace some of the other food? You can keep the same size plate and eat the same amount of food by weight, but just make it something like 40 percent protein, 40 percent carbohydrates and 20 percent vegetables.[25] If you are someone who cringes at the idea of eating vegetables on their own, because let's face it, a lot of them taste like sadness if you eat them plain, there are strategies for you to use beyond the obvious ones like becoming better with using seasonings to improve the flavor. For example, research has shown this effect can work even when you sneak hidden vegetables into other foods.[26] When I was a kid, I was a fussy little bugger and I hated onions, among other things. I would always pick them out of my dinner or eat around them. That's when my mum learned that if she chopped them so finely that I couldn't see them, it turns out I absolutely would eat onions after all. If hiding vegetables in dishes can work on children who are notorious for hating them,[27] it can probably work for you.

## Simplified Strategy to Reduce the Energy Density of Your Meals by Incorporating Fruits and Vegetables

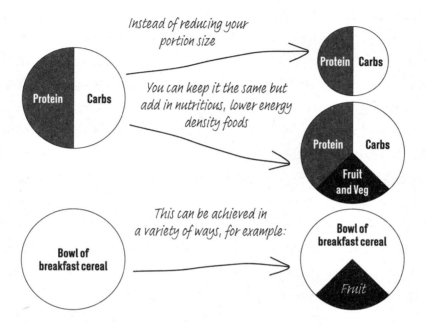

Alternatively, there is another strategy. Let's pretend you went to a food buffet. It is one of those all-you-can-eat places, so you intend to eat as much as you can to get your money's worth. What is one thing you definitely wouldn't do if your goal was to consume as much food as possible? Eat a salad. More specifically, eat a salad as a starter. Just the simple act of eating a salad first has been shown to reduce how much food you tend to eat at the subsequent main course.[28] The same thing has actually been shown with fruit as well—if you give people an apple to eat prior to serving them food, they will naturally eat less of their main dish.[29] Again, it is important to reiterate that these are tips that do not involve intentional calorie counting or dieting at all. They are just strategies that take advantage of your own appetite-control mechanisms so you naturally feel more full while eating more of the nutritious foods that most of us are already under-consuming, which sounds like a double win to me.

Here is another little-known fun fact. Although a lot of children hate eating vegetables, they will tend to be more receptive to eating them if they are served first in isolation without any more delicious competing foods. For example, if you give them carrots, broccoli or bell peppers to nibble on while they are waiting for lunch, they are likely to eat more of them than if you served the same vegetables alongside their main meal.[30,31] This actually works profoundly well on me, even in adulthood. I can remember precisely zero times in the past few years I have ever gone into the fridge to find a vegetable to nibble on because I am peckish between meals, but if there is a bowl of little tomatoes, carrot sticks or cucumber slices sitting in front of me while my dinner is cooking, I guarantee I will happily finish the whole thing.

Removing foods from your diet can feel like a fast-track ticket to pain and suffering. So it makes a nice change knowing you can add fruits and vegetables in and let them naturally displace other, more calorie-dense foods out of your diet. This comes with the added advantages of not requiring you to cut down your overall food intake by weight, avoiding the increased hunger you might experience from eating less, and improving the nutritional quality of your diet.

Adding vegetables to your diet can be expensive, especially if you pick fancy-sounding ones from exotic farmers' markets or high-end grocery stores, and this is one barrier to why many people don't eat enough.[32] If you fall into this camp, please rest assured knowing that the nutritional quality of frozen and even canned veggies is often very close to the fresh ones,[33,34] so eating more of these can be a very viable way to improve your diet at a more attractive price point.[35]

Here are some example goals and strategies for how you can easily eat more fruits and vegetables:

- As a starting point, you have probably heard of the classic "eat five a day" recommendation for servings of fruits and vegetables, and this appears to be a good ballpark for improved health benefits, if you do not include fruit juices and starchier vegetables like potatoes and corn.[36] Based on your own self-audit, you know if you have room for improvement, and maybe you don't need any strategies to implement this above and beyond this reminder.

- Allow fruits and vegetables to displace more calorie-dense foods from your main meals. For example, if you are eating fried chicken and chips (or fries for our American friends), adding in a side of vegetables can be a nutritious addition that naturally encourages you to consume fewer calories without realizing it and without even feeling hungrier. Likewise, if you are eating oatmeal, granola or another cereal, adding in chopped fruit can do the same thing as fruit tends to have a lower energy density than cereals and grains.

- If you are someone who doesn't love vegetables, chopping them up and hiding them in your meals can work extremely well because you often can't even taste them. For example, my wife can often squeeze two to three additional servings of veggies into a pasta sauce, stew or curry without me even noticing. I know this for a fact because we tested it. You can mix vegetables with rice dishes, blend them into meals with a sauce or add them into ground meat dishes like burgers and meatballs.

- Eating fruits and vegetables as a starter also works surprisingly well. If there is something you like the taste of, just having some in front of you when no other food is ready can prompt you to eat them without resentment, like me nibbling on mini tomatoes while I am cooking. My wife will often have a salad as a starter even when she isn't dieting because that's becoming her habitual way of eating more vegetables.

- Based on your self-audit, you already know if you are eating zero fruits and vegetables. In which case, feel free to aim for one to two per day first and, when you have that nailed, you can move on. Small changes can add up over time.

**Habit 3: Be mindful of extra dietary fat**

As we know from Chapter 3, lots of people are silly sausages and have very black-and-white views about foods. They view carbs and fats as either "good" or "bad," forgetting about all the shades of gray in the middle. I have seen hardcore low-carb fans talk about how healthy dietary fat is, while eating nothing but the cheese and pepperoni topping off a fast-food pizza or eating bacon and avocado slices deep fried in butter. There was even a trend for people to add several tablespoons of butter straight into their coffee. I am not even shitting you; these are real examples from people I have seen on social media. They believe that dietary fat is always great, and therefore you should eat it by the bucketload. Pro tip: there isn't really any food or drink that you can eat in unlimited quantities without harmful effects. Even drinking too much water can kill you, though it happens very rarely.

Dietary fats can be sneaky little buggers because they are often added into things without you even realizing it. People think that doughnuts and cookies are high-calorie and "bad" for you because of sugar, but both of these often contain more calories from fats than from sugars and carbohydrates. If you ever dare to try to make these without using lots of added oils or butter, you will quickly realize how important added fats are for texture and flavor.

Here is an example you will all recognize. Take a plain potato. If you bake it and eat it without any toppings, it tastes incredibly bland. What do restaurants do to make it taste better? They slather the humble potato with butter, bacon and cheese to make the mouthgasmic loaded potato. What do big food corporations do to make you more likely to buy their potatoes? They deep fry them in some kind of fat and turn them into crisps (chips) and French fries. The bland potato can become a delicious and somewhat addictive little fucker when you deep fry it enough. Part of the reason a lot of restaurant foods taste so good is because they drench things in a lot more butter and oil than you would use at home.

### Macronutrient Breakdown of Example Items at Popular Fast-Food Chains, by Calories

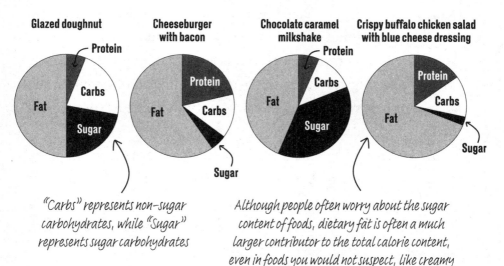

*"Carbs" represents non-sugar carbohydrates, while "Sugar" represents sugar carbohydrates*

*Although people often worry about the sugar content of foods, dietary fat is often a much larger contributor to the total calorie content, even in foods you would not suspect, like creamy milkshakes and even some chicken salads*

From our discussion on low-fat diets in Chapter 3, you now understand how they work. Fats are high in calories so removing higher-fat foods is a very quick way to reduce your calorie intake. I am not recommending you all suddenly go on an ultra-low-fat diet; I'm simply saying that you can reduce your intake of excessive amounts of dietary fat in general. It is estimated that over 70 percent of American adults exceed recommendations for eating saturated fat, and some of the most popular foods driving this are hot dogs, burgers, grilled cheese sandwiches and desserts.[37] In England, both children and adults are exceeding the recommended intake of saturated fat, on average, with the most common food contributors including things like biscuits, cakes, pastries and red meat.[38] If you are someone who really loves hot dogs, burgers, cakes and pastries, nobody is pointing a gun at your head saying you can never eat these ever again. Just keep in mind that it is possible for you to still eat them in exactly the same quantities with a reduced calorie content just by making some swaps, like choosing leaner cuts of meat or using reduced-fat dairy products.[39] You also don't need to eliminate all eggs, dairy and red meat from your diet, if you don't want to, as you can reduce your fat intake significantly simply by using easy tactics like grilling instead of frying,[40] and trimming excess fat off, which can sometimes reduce the amount of fat by over 50 percent.[41]

As a side note, people often have a misconstrued idea that any food that claims to be "lower in fat" is somehow unhealthier, because they must have replaced natural fat with dangerous additives, but that simply isn't the case. Lower-fat meat products are often just using leaner cuts, like comparing a higher-fat rib-eye steak to a leaner cut of filet mignon or a dark meat chicken thigh to a white meat chicken breast. Lower-fat dairy products are often just using skim milk instead of full-fat and don't always need more additives to make this switch. While it is true that some reduced-calorie and reduced-fat foods need formula changes, the most drastic ones tend to be in ultra-processed foods where they might add extra sugar, sweeteners or thickeners to help improve the taste and texture that removing some of the fat may have sacrificed. Reducing your intake of unnecessary additional dietary fats is not synonymous with eating "low-fat" versions of every single food, just like reducing your intake of excessive amounts of added sugar doesn't mean you should stop eating fruit where sugar is naturally occurring.

These are examples of why weight loss advice often includes "Eat reduced-fat foods where possible,"[42] but please keep in mind that this is not trying to tell you that all dietary fat is *bad*. You aren't supposed to have heart palpitations at the idea of cooking anything in oil, or eating anything with a higher fat content. Obviously, some foods that are high in fat can be problematic when consumed in large quantities, like eating huge amounts of saturated fat from processed red meat or a lot of oils from deep-fried foods, but many foods that are higher in fat are also linked with better health[43]—just like avocados, nuts and olive oil, which are commonly eaten in Mediterranean diets, are well known as a healthy dietary pattern (see page 69). It's just a smart idea to know that while dietary fat is important, it's also very easy to consume in excessive quantities without even realizing it.

Common examples of habit starting points include:

- Prioritize nutrient-dense, less processed foods over high-calorie, ultra-processed food, and there is a strong likelihood you will reduce your intake of added dietary fats as a by-product.

- Prioritize lean proteins over proteins very high in fat. Leaner proteins include white meat poultry like chicken and turkey breast, white fish and seafood like cod and shrimp, red meat with less visible fat, some Greek yogurts, legumes like chickpeas, and tofu, seitan and tempeh, which are popular for people avoiding animal products.
- Opt for grilling and air-frying over pan-frying and deep-frying, if you can do so without disproportionately sacrificing the taste of your meal, obviously.
- When eating very fatty cuts of red meat, consider trimming some of the excess off.
- If using a lot of sauces like dairy or mayonnaise, consider smaller portions or reduced-fat options as restaurant salad dressings that are creamy or cheesy can often be several hundred calories a go even for very small servings.
- Based on your own dietary audit, you have an idea of how you can move your own needle in a positive direction, so consider what you can do as painlessly as possible. Dietary fats are often stealthy creatures that we aren't always aware of even when we are eating excessive amounts of them. You absolutely shouldn't try to avoid them completely, but you might be surprised to realize how easy it is to make some little changes that add up to some substantial reductions if you are eating a lot of them.

### Habit 4: Prioritize lower-calorie drinks

If you go to your favorite big-chain coffee shop, you might notice that a lot of what they offer isn't really coffee anymore. You can get large frothy caramel macchiatos with extra syrup, whipped cream and marshmallows, if you fancy it. Now don't get me wrong, I am all for drinking something that feels like a dessert because life is short and who doesn't want to drink something that tastes like joy? A lot of the blended coffees tend to be in the region of a couple of hundred calories or so,[44] but in America, for example, it's not impossible for these coffee shop drinks to be made with heavy cream or ice cream and contain over 1,000 calories per serving. To put it into perspective, one of these drinks can easily be over half of some people's recommended total daily calorie intake. As we've discussed, these kinds of drinks didn't really exist even a few decades ago, so it's not surprising we are consuming more of our calories from drinks than we used to.[45] Super-high-calorie coffees might seem like an extreme example, but there are many less obvious examples of drinks that nudge up our energy intake, like milkshakes at fast-food restaurants or the abundance of sugary sodas that are sold in grocery stores, cafeterias, gas stations and vending machines.

Here's a fun fact. If you drink sugar in liquid form, it does not tend to fill you up as much as if you eat the same amount of sugar in solid form.[46] When bodybuilders want to gain weight and are struggling to consume enough food to really bulk up, it's quite common for them to turn to liquid nutrition as an easier way to consume more food than their appetite allows them to. I know because I have actually used this tactic myself even if I don't have the hulk-like physique to show for it. Liquid nutrition kind of bypasses the normal appetite mechanisms that make you feel full, so if you get in the habit of drinking more sugary drinks, these all tend to be additional calories on top of your regular diet.[47] If I gave you five oranges to eat in one go, it would take you several minutes to chew through them and you would probably feel full or get bored before you even peeled the final one. But it is super-duper easy to consume those same five oranges in the form of juice, and it would probably take you less than a minute to do so. Now take that concept and extend it to drinks made not only with refined sugar, but sometimes additional creams, syrups and ice cream.

Nobody thinks that eating a lot of ultra-processed, high-calorie sugary foods is a good idea, but drinking a lot of ultra-processed, high-calorie sugary drinks may actually be even worse for our health, because it's even easier to consume them in large quantities. This is why drinking a lot of sugary drinks is reliably linked with weight gain and worse health.[48] This is also why governments have tried stepping in to curtail the rising health risks, by implementing things like additional taxes on sugary drinks specifically.[49] This is kind of their way of saying, "Hey, we are really struggling to tell a whole country of people what they should eat, but if we make sugary drinks more expensive maybe people will switch back to water." Improving the health of a whole nation of people is extremely difficult, but you can at least tackle the most obvious culprits, like prohibiting teenagers from drinking alcohol and making cocaine completely illegal. Introducing taxes on sugary drinks is the middle ground way of trying to get us to drink them less often without banning them completely. Long story short: telling people to consume fewer liquid calories is one of the easiest, low-hanging-fruit ways of promoting weight loss.[50, 51, 52]

As always, you don't need to fully prohibit delicious higher-calorie drinks, if they float your boat. My wife loves putting creamer (a sweetened milk substitute) in her coffee and if someone told her she wasn't allowed to drink that anymore she would definitely tell that person to bugger off. Based on your own dietary audit, you know if there are any painless changes you would be happy to make.

## Health Risks Associated with Increased Intake of Sugar-Sweetened Beverages[53]

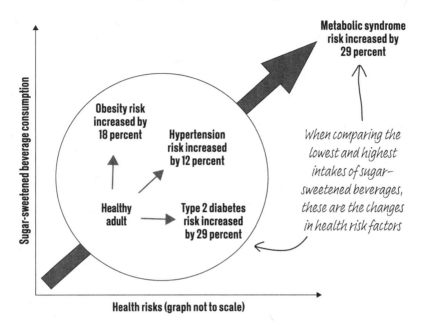

Here are some tips for prioritizing lower-calorie drinks:

- Prioritize water where possible. Nobody will ever argue against water being a great choice for a beverage, right?
- If you love sugary sodas, consider swapping for reduced-calorie versions, many of which can taste similar.
- If you enjoy sugary drinks (like fruit concentrate or "squash" as we call it in England), diluting it with more water is an easy way to decrease the energy density in each glass.
- If you enjoy high-calorie, more indulgent dessert-style coffees, try switching to lower-fat or lower-sugar creamers and sweeteners.
- Reduce alcohol intake, because alcohol can also be dangerous for your health for other reasons if you are consuming a lot.

## Habit 5: Exercise more, at least to a point

I know, I know, telling people it's a good idea to exercise is pointing out something so glaringly obvious that it runs the risk of feeling patronizing. That being said, it's important to know *why* we should exercise more, because most of us aren't doing enough of it. It's like brushing and flossing our teeth—we know it's a good thing, but our dentists still have to remind us in 101 different ways because they know most of us are shit at doing it twice a day like they keep nagging us to.

Regular physical exercise is linked with a decreased risk of over 25 chronic medical conditions including cardiovascular disease, type 2 diabetes and some cancers.[54] It also significantly reduces your all-cause mortality risk.[55] Obviously, we all die eventually, but if you look at big groups of people, those who exercise tend to live longer. If you look at elderly people specifically, the biggest modifiable predictors of how long they live include physical activity and physical function,[56] because being more mobile and stronger in your later years is always bound to be healthier than being frail and at a higher risk of injuring yourself. It's not just about physical health, either; exercise has been linked with better mental health, like reduced risk of depression in children and also adults.[57,58] If you want to stack the odds in your favor of being happier, healthier and living longer, it would be silly of you not to exercise.

Now here is the fun bit. You don't have to live in the gym to access this wonderful world of benefits. If anything, it seems like the biggest improvements to your health are seen at lower doses. If you currently do absolutely fuck all exercise and you spend the entirety of your days lying on the couch, you can reap huge benefits from doing a moderate amount of exercise. On the flip side, someone who already trains a lot may not get anything from training more. You will do more for your health by going from 0 to 50 than someone will likely get by going from 50 to 100.

### Theoretical Dose–Response Relationship Between Physical Activity/Fitness and Health Status[59]

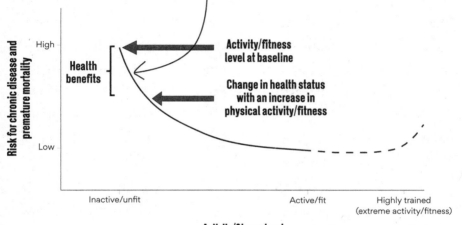

*Although being super fit can obviously be good for your health, significant health improvements can also be seen at much lower thresholds, so doing something will likely always be better for your health than doing nothing!*

Something crucially important to understand is that exercising a little bit more in isolation is not always a reliable way to lose weight unless you also pair it with nutrition changes, or at least make sure you keep your food intake static. There are possibly three big reasons for this.

Firstly, exercising actually doesn't tend to burn as many calories as most people think. Let's say Bobbie the Beginner wants to lose some weight, so they decide to join the gym and start jogging. As Bobbie is brand new to working out, it's fair to say their jogging is at quite a gentle pace, because diving headfirst from a sedentary sofa lifestyle immediately into a speedy treadmill sprint would be a great recipe for pulling a hamstring or having a heart attack, both of which are not ideal. Depending on their age, how much they weigh and a load of other factors, Bobbie is probably going to burn in the region of a couple of hundred extra calories per jog.[60] But let's be generous and round up to 500. If they jog two or three times per week, that is in the ballpark of 1,000–1,500 calories. It is commonly estimated that women require 2,000 calories per day and men 2,500 calories per day just to maintain their weight, although again this depends on a metric shit-ton of factors. That means that a typical woman and a typical man are burning 14,000 to 17,500 calories per week. Doing some very quick math, that means, out of all the energy Bobbie is burning every week, less than 10 percent actually comes from exercising. In fact, for an average person, it's estimated that only around 5 percent of the energy you burn comes from working out.[61] Of course, if you work out spleen-bustingly hard or for very long periods of time this will make a difference, but that is not most people.

Secondly, exercising a lot can make some people disproportionately hungry. If you go for a jog and burn a couple of hundred calories but your appetite also goes up a little bit and your body craves more than a couple of hundred calories of food, any calorie burn effect of the exercise gets wiped out. Have you ever left the gym and felt like you needed to grab an extra chocolate bar on the way out because you felt ravenous? Well, that. This phenomenon does not happen to everyone, but it is well observed in research literature that people who start exercising more often do not get the weight loss results they expect and a subset of people actually gain weight when they start exercising more.[62,63,64]

Thirdly, exercising a lot can make you move less elsewhere. If you finish your jog and suddenly feel like you need to spend the rest of the day on the sofa, you are increasing your physical activity via exercise but then reducing it in your daily life. This is referred to as a "constrained" model of exergy expenditure, which basically just means the calories you burned in the gym are not purely additive to how many you burn normally. Although the magnitude of it is up for debate,[65,66,67] the concept is something worth being aware of.

While exercising can indeed be useful as a fat loss tool, that is contingent on other factors that most people are not aware of. It is extremely common for people to start going to the gym with the sole goal of losing weight, but then feel discouraged when they don't get the results they expect.[68]

This is very important to understand because I would absolutely love it if you made exercise part of your regular routine, for the rest of your life. I don't want you just to do it to see the number on the scales going down and then give up when that inevitably stops happening. Remember, nobody can continually lose weight forever without literally dying, which is definitely suboptimal. That being said, even if the scales are unable to show you all the benefits of exercising, exercise can still change your actual body composition. For example, it can be particularly beneficial for reducing visceral fat,[69,70] which is deep fat stored around your organs—the kind of thing you cannot see just by stepping on the scales, but a health risk factor if you have a lot of it.[71] Even though not everyone who exercises more will suddenly see a lot of weight loss, some people do, and it can also be good for promoting fat loss and helping hold on to precious muscle tissue when dieting.[72]

If you had an identical twin and both of you weighed the exact same amount, but you exercised, had a lower body fat percentage, had more muscle mass and had lower levels of visceral fat, you would expect to be the healthier twin. So, judging how useful exercise is based solely on whether you lose weight or not is a bit like judging how useful your legs are solely by whether you can do backflips or not. It ignores many wonderful benefits and zooms in on one that tends to be less important, unless your career revolves around doing backflips, of course. In an ideal world, exercise should not be an attractive thing you have a short-term fling with before getting bored and moving on. It should be the kind of thing you want to spend the rest of your life with and that's why it's important to try to find a form of exercise you enjoy enough to keep repeating forever.

Here are some good starting points for introducing more exercise into your life:

- In an ideal world, perform 150–300 minutes of moderate-intensity or 75–150 minutes of vigorous-intensity aerobic exercise per week, and do muscle-strengthening activities, like weight training, at least twice per week. These are the standard recommendations on improving your health from institutions like the WHO.[73] However, please consider these as delightful long-term targets because they are universally prescribed for everyone, not customized for your own individual circumstances. Based on your own self-audit, that might be a very distant destination from where you are now, in which case don't be disheartened if it looks like it is beyond the horizon. Feel reassured that moving toward that destination at all is going to be a great thing for your health.
- For example, if you are currently doing 20 minutes of aerobic work twice per week, there are several ways you can move the needle in a positive direction. You could increase your workout frequency

to three times per week or more. You could increase your duration from 20 to 25 minutes or more. You could also increase the intensity of your workouts so you maximize the efficiency of those 20-minute periods without extending the workout period itself.

- For resistance training specifically, this does not have to be gym-focused. Doing body-weight exercises can be a great starting point until you feel more comfortable using additional weights, and this can often be enough to help hold on to precious muscle tissue when dieting, especially if you are a beginner.

### Habit 6: Increase lifestyle activity

When it comes to fat loss, most people immediately default to thinking about what exercise routine they should start following, but here is the thing most people don't realize: your body actually burns more energy keeping you alive and moving around in daily life than it does from a typical workout. You are burning energy all the time, even if you are doing absolutely nothing. You can lie in bed all day watching the TV and your heart is still beating, your lungs are still breathing and your organs are still functioning. You may have heard the term "resting metabolic rate" or "basal metabolic rate," which just means how much energy your body burns naturally even when you aren't doing anything. Once you eat food, your body burns a bit more energy digesting that food and, as soon as you roll over in bed or get up and walk to the bathroom, your body burns more energy again. So, out of all the things you do that burn energy, exercising is not the biggest contributor. The biggest contributor that you are actually in control of is something called "non-exercise activity thermogenesis" or "NEAT." This is a very fancy term for energy burned through all movement outside of intentional exercise. All those little things you do throughout the course of the day, like walking, climbing stairs, carrying shopping bags, typing on your laptop, fidgeting at your desk and scratching your butt crack when nobody is looking, they all burn a teeny tiny bit of energy, which can accumulate to a lot.

For example, if you have a highly physical job, you could be burning a whopping 2,000 calories per day or more compared to your hypothetical twin who has a sedentary job,[74] which is probably at least four times more than Bobbie burned during their gentle treadmill jog we talked about earlier. This is why so many researchers actually say the key to weight management probably isn't about hyper-focusing on how active you are in the gym, but instead shifting your attention to its neglected sibling: how active you are in your day-to-day life.[75,76,77]

## How Your Body Burns Energy[78]

- Exercise (exercise activity thermogenesis or EAT): Energy burned from working out. For most, this is surprisingly small.
- Non-exercise activity thermogenesis (NEAT): Energy burned through all other physical movement outside of exercise. This is neglected, but usually more significant than exercise itself.
- Thermic effect of food (TEF): Additional energy burned when you eat food. This goes up if you significantly increase your calorie intake and down if you reduce it. What you eat can also influence this, but it is a relatively small contributor to overall energy burn.
- Basal metabolic rate (BMR): Energy burned just staying alive. This is primarily dictated by your body size and composition, so it increases when you gain weight and decreases when you lose weight. It can also go up a teeny bit if you build more muscle.

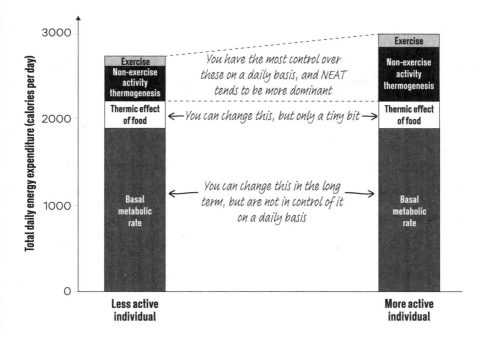

Now here is the pickle. In some ways, squeezing the gym into your schedule might be easier as you can do quick 30-minute workouts, but our overall lifestyles are slowly making it harder to remain active on a day-to-day basis. Many of us work long hours sitting on our arses in sedentary desk jobs, have to rely on cars for transportation instead of walking or cycling, and get our shopping delivered to us to save us the time and effort of walking around the stores. Therefore, significantly increasing your daily physical movement outside of exercising is often dependent on the cumulation of very small behaviors, rather than one big one.

Here are some example habits for increasing lifestyle activity:

- The most common recommendation is for you to walk at least 10,000 steps per day, because it's an easy-to-remember, nice round number, and people who walk more often lose weight and improve their health.[79,80] Double win. But that's actually a fuckload of steps and can be very hard to achieve if you don't spend a lot of the day on your feet. So, if your current activity levels are very low, please know that walking a little bit more may decrease your risk of dying early, even if you do fewer than 10,000 steps a day.[81,82] Based on your own self-audit you have an idea of how active you are, so do what you can to move the needle upward at an appropriate pace.

- On top of that, it's a great idea to build movement into your daily life, where possible. For example, can you use a standing desk instead of a seated desk, take your calls standing up instead of sitting down, take the stairs instead of the escalator, park farther away from the entrance to the grocery store, take short breaks from working at your desk, get outside or do something after dinner rather than sitting on the couch, and so on?

## Nonlinear Dose–Response Analyses of Step Count and Risk of All-Cause Mortality[83]

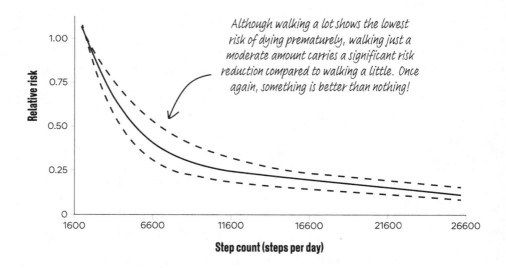

Although walking a lot shows the lowest risk of dying prematurely, walking just a moderate amount carries a significant risk reduction compared to walking a little. Once again, something is better than nothing!

### Habit 7: Exercise snacks

Just to really drive home the point that doing some form of physical activity is better than doing nothing, there is a growing amount of research on something called "exercise snacking." If a gym workout is a big meal, an exercise snack is a very short duration of physical activity that you might do multiple times per day. These snacks might be teeny tiny, as short as 60 seconds long,[84] or they might be a little smidge more substantial, like 2–5 minutes long.[85]

The simplified idea here is, a lot of people are really fucking struggling to hit the proposed activity guidelines, as you already know from reading this book. Rather than people missing out on all the delicious benefits that exercise can provide, can they get a little taste of those benefits just from doing a little bit of exercise? Doing one to five minutes of exercise might sound pathetic to people who work out a lot, but it does possibly have a wonderful upside: it is easier to squeeze into your routine. Driving to and from the gym can take time, so rather than doing nothing, you can try exercise snacks. By starting small and being consistent, this could allow you to build a habit into your routine (yay) and make it easier to do something called "habit stacking," which is piggybacking a new behavior onto an existing behavior.

I used to work with a fellow personal trainer and, when the unpredictable English summer rolled around (all two weeks of it), he came into work wearing a pair of shorts and I noticed how much more muscular his calves were since the last time I saw them. He laughed and said, "Mate, do you know what my secret is? I do calf raises every time I brush my teeth. That's it." As brushing his teeth is a habit that he spends a few minutes each day doing, he stacked the habit of doing calf raises at the same time, and he was very happy with the results.

Small habits performed consistently can accumulate. Do you ever sit on the toilet, get out your phone and send messages or emails? Well, replying to work emails for five minutes obviously isn't as productive as sitting at your computer for eight hours like a full day of work, but if you did it several times per day it is significantly better than sending zero emails at all. That's how exercise snacks work. On social media in 2024 I started promoting something called "60-Second Movement." This was just an open invitation for anyone to start a new habit for one single measly minute at a time. Some people from around the world joined in by doing things like using a jump rope, performing yoga or doing push-ups. Even though one minute sounds feeble, it acts as a gateway to test a new behavior, get better at it and hopefully increase your enjoyment, which then allows you to be consistent. Even within the first 30 days of the free challenge I saw total strangers getting significantly better at their chosen activity, which is evidence of the power of tiny habits performed consistently.

Let me be crystal clear: doing a couple of minutes of exercise per day isn't suddenly going to transform the way your physique looks, feels or functions, regardless of how hard you work during those times. But a few minutes performed multiple times per day could accumulate toward 15–30 minutes of exercise daily, and that is substantial enough to make a difference. While the research is new, exercise snacks do have the power to improve your health, like your cardiorespiratory fitness levels,[86] and people with higher fitness levels do tend to live longer.[87] So, if you are struggling to squeeze exercise into your routine already, or there are certain aspects of a fitness regimen that you are neglecting, here are some ideas of how exercise snacks could help you:

- In theory, interrupting sedentary time by doing anything less sedentary is always going to be a win, hence why one of the habits we mentioned earlier was simply to stand up for ten minutes for every hour you spend sitting down.[88]

- Depending on your abilities, preferences and circumstances, you can do things like running up and down the stairs, brief stints of just walking around, or do some body-weight exercises. Needless to say, these should enrich your life, and should not be seen as a stressful way of squeezing in some exercise. Please don't become that obsessive person who needs to do sets of push-ups in the bathroom of a restaurant or nightclub (which a friend of mine has genuinely seen before).

- Pairing exercise snacks with something you already do in daily life can help reinforce the subconscious nature of habit building. There are some things you already do every day, like brushing your teeth, making a coffee or waiting for your shower to heat up before you hop in, that might give you a good opportunity to habit stack.

- Exercise snacks don't have to be used as a way of starting exercise from scratch, they can also be used as a way to incorporate neglected forms of exercise. For example, I lift weights a lot, but I have spent a lot of my life neglecting my aerobic fitness, so I started doing one to three minutes of skipping (or jumping rope, as they call it in America) after my regular workouts, as a quick way of bundling on something that would improve my fitness levels to something that I already did as part of my ingrained routine.

## Habit 8: Ensure adequate sleep quality

You know when you are really sleep-deprived and your body just starts feeling like absolute dog shit? You feel tired all the time, your motivation to do anything decreases and your brain sharpness starts feeling less like a knife, and more like a blunt teaspoon. We all instinctively know that good-quality sleep is important for our physical and mental health, right? Although it is a tricky thing to study over the long term, it is not surprising that sleep duration and sleep quality are likely linked with a shit-ton of health conditions, including all-cause mortality.[89]

What many people do not know is that poor sleep quality can also impact your body weight and body fat specifically. One aspect of this is that, when you are sleep-deprived, your body can experience hormonal changes that make you feel hungrier.[90] Have you ever noticed that if you haven't been getting much sleep, you are more inclined to lie in a near-vegetative state on the couch and your brain feels more snack-curious than it does normally? Well, that. The extra surprising thing is that you don't need to get terrible sleep for months for this to happen; these hormonal shifts could start occurring after just one single night of sleep deprivation.[91,92] For example, in one study of just a single night of sleep deprivation, people who only slept for 4 hours instead of 8 consumed 559 more calories (22 percent more food) the following day.[93] On top of this, people who were sleep-deprived seemed to have an increased preference for high-fat foods. It's quite possible that being exhausted doesn't just make you want to eat more, but eat more high-calorie less nutritious foods specifically.[94] If I think back about the times I am really tired, I always fancy munching on a bag of cookies, but never touch the bag of carrots we almost always have in our fridge.

## Calorie Intake Following One Night of Different Sleep Durations[95]

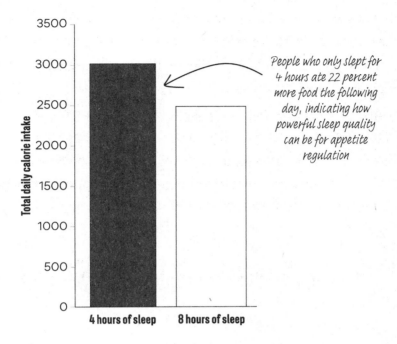

*People who only slept for 4 hours ate 22 percent more food the following day, indicating how powerful sleep quality can be for appetite regulation*

And if that sounds startling, it actually gets worse. Sleep deprivation not only makes you inclined to eat more food, but it can also make you more susceptible to losing muscle tissue when you are dieting. One study compared short 14-day periods of either 8.5 or 5.5 hours of sleep in the context of a reduced-calorie diet and, although both conditions resulted in the same weight loss, sleep deprivation caused less fat loss and more lean body mass loss.[96] So, if you and your identical twin were both following an identical diet and lost an identical amount of weight, but you were sleep-deprived and they weren't, your weight loss would likely come more from muscle tissue and less from fat tissue than their weight loss, which is not ideal.

This sounds like fucking terrible news, but it also means that the reverse is true. You can actually regulate your appetite, improve your diet, increase muscle tissue retention and increase fat loss as a downstream effect of improving your sleep quality. If you are habitually sleep-deprived and you manage to increase your sleep duration, it's quite likely that you will naturally reduce how much food you are eating without even trying. In another study, people who received sleep counseling to extend their sleep by just over one hour per night naturally consumed 270 fewer calories compared to those who carried on with their usual sleep patterns[97]—no dieting, no intentional food restriction; your body's appetite hormones may simply settle after being out of whack for a while, so you crave food less.

**Change in Calorie Intake (calories per day) During the 2-Week Intervention[98]**

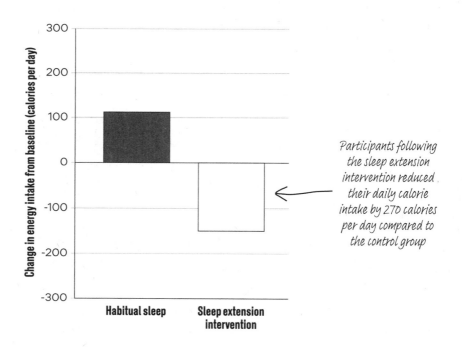

Participants following the sleep extension intervention reduced their daily calorie intake by 270 calories per day compared to the control group

Not only that, but you can also improve your body composition changes as well. So, if you and your twin now followed exactly the same exercise program, but you were smart, you read this book and then decided to implement some sleep optimization tips, you could actually lose more body fat than your twin would, as demonstrated in research.[99]

Below are some sleep optimization tips you can implement. The goal would be to practice these consistently, so they become habitual behaviors you can reap the rewards from.

### Sleep optimization tips[100]

- Keep it dark, quiet and cool in the room you sleep in.
- Go to bed and wake up at the same time of the day, including weekends.
- Go to bed at a time that allows you eight hours of sleep.
- Try to get enough sleep so you do not need to rely on an alarm clock.
- Avoid strong caffeine sources like energy drinks and coffee within six hours of bedtime.
- Learn a relaxation technique that helps you fall asleep.

Two hours before bed:

- Turn down the lights.
- Minimize use of electronic devices, or use the lowest light settings, because staring at a bright phone screen two inches from your eyeballs isn't super peaceful for your brain.
- Avoid exercise.

- Avoid tea, or any other drinks with caffeine, even if the caffeine content is lower.
- Do calm and positive activities. Avoid arguing with your partner, which might just be a sensible life rule in general.

When you wake up in the morning:

- Expose yourself to as much light as possible right away, because staying in a pitch-black cave for a long time when you wake up isn't super conducive to feeling alert, given that light and darkness are powerful influencers of your internal biological clock that can help regulate your sleep patterns.

Obviously, not everyone has the luxury of having long, restful and uninterrupted sleep. If you are an insomniac, shift worker or parent of a beautiful yet incessantly screaming child, someone telling you to "just get eight hours of sleep a night"—as if that's an easy thing for you to achieve—may make you want to give them a frustrated flick to the forehead. That being said, if you can see some easy things from the sleep optimization tips above for you to work on, these could help promote better appetite regulation, weight loss and fat loss without you having to work harder. In a world of fad diets and aggressive ways of restricting your food intake, improving your sleep patterns is a refreshingly healthy habit that can have a huge impact on your overall health, well-being and body composition as a consequence.

### Habit 9: Consume adequate protein

You already know from Chapter 3 that eating more protein can help promote fat loss and aid muscle retention when dieting, which is a double win (see page 66). Now I would like to talk about something slightly different: appetite. Some people say that protein is the most filling macronutrient, and I think that's a bit of an exaggeration. Saying protein makes you feel fuller than carbohydrates and fats implies that *all* protein foods are better at making you feel full than *all* carbohydrates and *all* fats. While eating a big portion of chicken or steak might satisfy your hunger for a few hours longer than eating some gummy worms, drinking a liquid protein shake probably wouldn't do the same thing, and that protein shake is unlikely to fill you up better than a serving of oatmeal or potatoes. How satisfied you feel after eating something is a lot more complex than the macronutrient content of that meal alone. Protein can play a role, but just how much of a role is a tricky thing to say for sure.[101]

That being said, here is a simple example of the role that protein might play. How do you feel when you wake up, then treat yourself to a muffin, a pastry or a bowl of sugary cereal for breakfast before going to work? A lot of typical breakfast foods are high in sugar, ultra-processed to be extra delicious, and often not that great for appetite regulation compared to less processed foods with a lower energy density. So, there is a strong possibility you might start feeling peckish a couple of hours later and turn into a little snack goblin searching for a tasty treat to keep you going.

Some research has shown that if you give teenagers lower-protein, higher-sugar breakfast meals like oatmeal sweetened with sugar, they will feel significantly hungrier afterward than they do if they eat higher-protein, lower-sugar breakfast meals like an omelet with fresh fruit. This hunger difference was so large in fact that, at their next meal, they ate 81 percent more food.[102] This shows the power that the first meal can have on the rest of your day. If you feel hungry as fuck and your body naturally wants you to eat more food, it doesn't take a genius to realize that this can make dieting harder. This might also work with other foods, like eating eggs for breakfast instead of a bagel.[103] In fact, if you take people who skip breakfast and give them a high-protein breakfast instead, this might help their appetite management so much that it could promote weight loss over skipping breakfast completely.[104]

The most important protein variable for fat loss, muscle growth and appetite regulation is probably just consuming enough in general, and how often you eat it matters far less. For example, if someone is not consuming enough protein and they increase their daily intake, this will have a much more powerful impact than if they decide to split that protein intake over two, three, four or however many meals they fancy per day. The research on this is quite mixed, and it definitely is not as straightforward as, "If you eat more protein for breakfast, you will definitely feel less hungry and definitely lose a lot of weight."[105,106] But, I think it is a very smart idea for you to experiment with different breakfasts to see how you feel. For example, I have a soft spot for chocolaty cereal that's definitely marketed to kids rather than adults. If I eat a bowl of that sugary deliciousness for breakfast, I can bet good money I will feel hungry again a couple of hours later. However, if I make oatmeal and add some protein to it, like protein powder or a protein-rich yogurt, my appetite levels are way lower over the course of the day, especially if I also combine fruit (like the energy density displacement strategies we discussed earlier). Also, we know that it is common for people not to eat that much protein in the morning, and consume most of it later in the day, so adding more to breakfast might be a sensible strategy to make sure you are eating enough in general.[107]

Based on your own self-audit, if you think you notice you have a lot of meals without a source of protein, here are some example habit starting points:

- For fat loss and muscle growth, consuming more protein can be useful. Foods that contain protein include meat, fish, seafood, dairy, eggs, soy products, beans and lentils. The most important thing is consuming enough in general, and how often you eat it matters far less.

- However, knowing that it can have a role to play in how hungry you feel, a common dietary tip is prioritizing protein at breakfast specifically, which has the power to help regulate your appetite levels throughout the day. This can be very beneficial given a lot of people don't consume much protein in the morning, and also tend to eat a lot more food in the evening, especially if they have let their hunger build up.

- Alternatively, it can be a good idea to just make sure you are consuming a source of protein at all of your main meals. This is a decent ballpark behavioral recommendation for gaining or retaining muscle tissue while dieting and, although it isn't magic for appetite regulation, if you try it and notice it helps with your energy levels and how satisfied you feel after meals, that is a great thing to find out. Play around and see what works for you.

## Habit 10: Eat without distractions

Have you ever sat down in front of your favorite TV show or film, opened a pack of your favorite snacks and a couple of minutes later realized that you have plowed your way through the whole thing without even realizing it? I know it can't just be me, but if I sit down in a movie theater with some popcorn or candy, there's a solid possibility that I will have scarfed it all down before the trailers have even finished, barely pausing to savor the flavor.

For many years, scientists have noted a relationship between television watching and body weights. For example, children and adolescents who watch a lot of TV tend to weigh more and have a higher risk of obesity.[108] Obviously, this might simply be because kids who watch several hours of TV every day are also sitting down a lot, which implies they have a sedentary lifestyle. It is also complicated by the fact that TV programs often feature delicious food commercials and product placements, which can subconsciously nudge people toward eating more food, like we discussed earlier (see page 24).[109,110]

It's also been shown that, if you are watching TV, you may naturally gravitate toward eating more food simply because TV serves as a distraction from what you are putting in your mouth. In one study, adults were given the same meal of macaroni and cheese or pizza and were allowed to pick a program of their choice to watch. During a 30-minute episode, participants watching TV ate 71 percent more mac and cheese and 36 percent more pizza than they did when they were listening to music instead.[111] As it turns out, if you eat food in front of your favorite show, you may eat it significantly quicker than you would normally and this is a solid recipe for getting more food into you before you feel full.

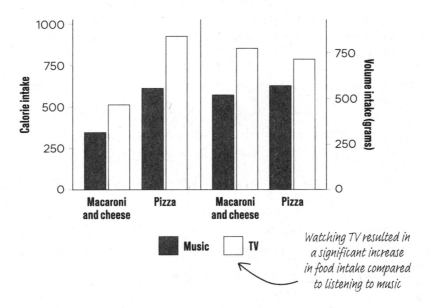

### Calorie Intake and Food Volume Intake While Watching TV or Listening to Music[112]

Watching TV resulted in a significant increase in food intake compared to listening to music

If you eat a lot more during a mere 30-minute TV episode, imagine what could happen if you are someone who eats all of your dinners and evening snacks in front of the TV. Over the course of weeks, months, years or decades that could really tally up. This distracted eating concept isn't only applicable to the TV. If your boss is an arsehole who makes you feel guilty for taking lunch breaks, so you eat while you are working on your laptop,[113] or you are someone who likes playing on your smartphone while you are snacking,[114] it's quite possible that this is naturally pushing you toward eating more food without you even realizing it. In today's fast-paced, technology-fueled environment, these types of distractions are all around us, and they may interfere with your body's natural ability to tell you when you have eaten enough food. This is why avoiding distractions while you are eating may be a smart way to be more in-tune with your body's natural hunger signals, which often means you will end up eating less food without having to count calories, monitor your portion sizes, or any of that shit.[115]

Here are some example habits for eating without distractions:

- If you are someone who notices that your snack hand speeds up while you are watching TV or playing on your phone or computer, it might be a good idea to eat your meals elsewhere, like at a dining table or separate desk. You can of course watch TV afterward, but separating it away from when you eat might be smart.
- If you are like me and my wife, and you notice that, when you are tired, you find yourself mindlessly watching your favorite show surrounded by an array of delicious snacks, sometimes it's a good idea to turn off the TV and do something else.
- Alternatively, be smarter with your snack selection, of course.

**Habit 11: Slow down when you eat**

While we are on the topic of eating while distracted, there is another pro tip that overlaps with this. Returning to the analogy of the all-you-can-eat buffet, imagine you really wanted to get your money's worth. What strategy would you have if your goal was to cram as much food into you as you physically could before your stomach eventually said, "OK, stop being a dickhead, I have had more than enough for today"? You would eat quickly. Subconsciously, I think most of us already know this, right? Let's say you visit the exact same buffet on two separate occasions, and you can eat as much food as you want on both:

Visit 1: You chew each mouthful of food at least 20 times to savor the flavor, you pause between mouthfuls and put your knife and fork back on the plate. If you want to refill your plate you wait at least five minutes after finishing your last one.

Visit 2: You barely chew each mouthful and swallow it as quickly as your pending indigestion allows. Before you have even swallowed, you already have your next mouthful on your fork going into your mouth. When your plate is finished you immediately get up to refill it before you have even swallowed the mouthful you are still chewing.

In both scenarios, you could have exactly the same food selection in front of you, but we both know that you would be able to eat far more food on your second visit than your first. The theory is, there are certain appetite signals that your stomach will send to your brain to tell you that you are full, so if you have the goal of stuffing as much food into your body as possible, you need to do it quickly before these appetite signals kick in. Some research has found a link between how fast you eat and the risk of metabolic syndrome and obesity.[116,117] In simple terms, people who eat faster often tend to weigh more and people who eat slower often tend to weigh less.

If I am in a movie theater and eating popcorn, my natural inclination is to use my hand as a kind of makeshift shovel, dive it into the box and pick up as much as I can before throwing it vaguely at my mouth. Most of it will go in and, while I am chewing, my shovel hand is already ready to go again. If I intentionally slowed down how fast I ate, it is quite likely that I would naturally eat less of that popcorn.[118] Not because I am calorie counting, not because I have measured out a measly portion of it to ration out, but simply because I wasn't racing to stuff as much as possible into my mouth before my appetite signals kicked in. If you feel like you are someone who eats food rapidly and mindlessly, being conscious of slowing things down a bit, using the tips I am about to provide, might be a smart idea. Something I notice a lot when traveling is that in healthier Mediterranean cultures, people tend to eat much slower and mealtimes are often long and drawn out. Lunch can last two to three hours, with long breaks between courses. This is in stark contrast to a lot of American restaurants where food tends to be served very quickly and you might be in and out in less than 30 minutes.

Practice the following to help slower eating habits become your norm:

- If, like me, you eat quickly and barely chew before swallowing, try chewing for longer and focus on savoring each mouthful. This shouldn't be a stressful practice, and don't do anything silly like trying to chew each mouthful one hundred times, because that sounds like a rapid way to ruin how much you enjoy your meal.
- Put your cutlery down or pause between mouthfuls.
- Have longer pauses between courses. If you start eating dessert within milliseconds of finishing your main meal, you are naturally going to want to eat more of it than if there was a gap, even if you are enjoying exactly the same dessert.

### Habit 12: Engineer your immediate food environment

For a moment, I want you to imagine your favorite snack. Pause to think about it for a second. Personally, I really love warm cookies.

Something about the gooey chocolate chips really revs my engine and adding a scoop of cold ice cream for good measure makes this even more fucking delicious. Now, whatever your favorite snack is, I want you to imagine that I put it right in front of you as you read this book. You can see it and you might even be able to smell it. Unless you are a biological anomaly, there is a strong possibility that this snack is going to start subconsciously calling your name. You might not fancy it right now, but by the time you turn a few pages, you already know it is probably going to be snack time.

This is the power that your immediate food environment can have on your food cravings. You might not be hungry when you start shopping in the grocery store, but there is a reason that the bakery they have in the corner pumps the smell of freshly baked bread and cookies into the aisles. It can take you from a zero to a ten on the snack-curious scale in the blink of an eye.

As we've explored earlier, research shows that you tend to eat foods that are most convenient to you (see page 18). If a snack is placed within arm's reach, you are more likely to eat it than if it was on the other side of the table.[119] So, if you work in an office that always has doughnuts in the kitchen, all it takes is for one of your colleagues to move those doughnuts to your desk so they are within arm's reach and suddenly you are much more likely to be eating doughnuts for lunch. This is also one of the many ways grocery stores can secretly manipulate your purchasing patterns. For example, when you are standing in line for the checkout, you are within convenient grabbing distance of a lot of snacks, which are there to make it as easy as possible for you to add them to your basket. Now, here is the interesting bit. This same behavioral mechanism actually has the potential to be a force for good when properly harnessed. If grocery stores gave a fuck about your health rather than their profits, they could encourage consumption of more nutritious food options simply by making them more convenient.[120] For example, if the snack sections near the checkouts stopped selling soda and started selling water instead, or they stopped selling candy and started selling fruit and nuts, you would subconsciously be more inclined to buy the more nutritious options instead without even realizing it.[121,122] Grocery stores can also steer you away from buying alcohol, one of the most agreed upon dangerous types of drink to consume in excess, simply by not advertising it on the large, end-of-aisle promotional displays.[123]

So, here is how I would like you to think about it. If you put a handheld games console in front of a child, they are probably going to want to play on that games console, right? It's convenient and fun to play, and now it's got their attention. But once they have it, you can't just snatch the games console away without running the risk of them throwing a tantrum because you prohibited their favorite treat. So, it might be a better idea to replace it with something more favorable instead. Multiple research studies support the idea of making nutritious foods more convenient to increase your likelihood of eating them.[124] In today's modern environment, you are increasingly surrounded by tasty treats that are high-calorie, extra delicious and cheaper to buy than ever, which makes resisting these foods extremely difficult.[125] Rather than telling yourself that you cannot eat any of the delicious foods that you encounter in day-to-day life, which is probably an express train ticket to feeling deprived and miserable, make preferred choices more convenient to decrease the amount of mental willpower you need to exert to make that choice. This goes back to the concept we discussed earlier of habit substitution versus abrupt habit discontinuation (see page 119). Not eating a chocolate bar when it's the only food choice right in front of you and you are feeling peckish might be really fucking hard, but if you don't have chocolate in the house or the chocolate bar is hidden away in the pantry cupboard and an apple is in front of you, you are far more likely to eat the apple and less likely to eat the chocolate than you would have been before. The goal is to reduce the friction of making positive choices to make it easier on yourself.

To make healthy food choices habitual, try the following suggestions to take control of your immediate food environment:

- Based on your self-audit, you can identify when your prime less-than-nutritious snacking opportunities occur and try to make your preferred choices more convenient, like taking fruit to work and keeping it on your desk instead of relying on snacks from the vending machine.

- Position ideal choices at the front of your fridge and pantry cupboards so they are more visible and accessible. If your most convenient foods aren't the ones you want to be eating regularly, you are putting yourself in a position where you have to work harder to swim upstream to get the same result.

- If you know there are times when you often resort to less nutrient-dense, high-calorie fast-food options, for example, when you are tired, make sure you have equally fast nutritious options on hand—something you can eat quickly when you are hungry or exhausted. If a nutritious meal takes 30 minutes to cook and a less nutritious meal takes just a couple of minutes to cook, there is bound to be more friction to eating the more nutritious meal.

- You can also engineer your immediate environment to make other healthier choices. For example, position your gym clothes somewhere you will see them as an easy visual reminder to do your exercise for the day. Keep your smartphone out of the bedroom at night to ensure you get a restful night's sleep instead of succumbing to the temptation of keeping yourself awake by doomscrolling at 1am.

### Habit 13: Keep a regular eating pattern

How many meals you eat per day actually makes surprisingly little difference to how much body fat you lose. What I mean by this is, if you take your day's worth of food and lay it out on a table in front of you, you can divide that however you want, into as many meals or as few meals as you please. You could eat it all in two big meals, or divide it into nine teeny-tiny meals, and as long as your total food intake stays the same, then the difference it makes is probably less than a smidge above absolutely fuck all.[126]

But it *can* make a difference, if changing your meal frequency causes you to eat fewer calories as a by-product—as in the example of intermittent fasters who often eat less food as a consequence of skipping breakfast (see page 80).

Although there isn't a perfect number of meals you all need to strive for, maintaining a regular eating pattern by eating at the same times each day can be beneficial for other reasons. For example, if you have a really sporadic eating schedule and on some days you find your snacking going through the roof as a consequence of that, keeping a regular meal rhythm might be useful to decrease your snacking habit.[127] Likewise, if you go for long periods of time without food and then you feel so hungry that you end up binge eating afterward, having a snack earlier in the day might be a beneficial thing, which is why three meals per day plus two to three planned snacks is often recommended to decrease binge-eating episodes.[128]

I have had the pleasure of looking through many food diaries in my time, and talking to countless clients, and if you asked me to bet money on the meals that most people feel like they have a problem with, I would place all that money on two meal types: evenings and weekends. It is incredible to see how common it is for people to feel like they are dieting successfully most of the time, but their evenings and weekends feel like they are out of control. If you work a 9 to 5 job, there is a decent chance that your 9 to 5 diet is fairly routine, but then, after 5pm, the metaphorical train comes off the tracks and feels like it smashes into a hedge. Sometimes the train runs a pretty normal schedule during the week, but then, at the weekend, it's not just a hedge that it crashes into, but a fiery oblivion. One research study in highly successful dieters concluded that people who dieted consistently during the whole week were more likely to successfully maintain their weight loss than people who dieted even more strictly during the week and less strictly at the weekend.[129] However, it can also go too far in the other direction because trying to be extremely strict all the time can be counterproductive. Another study found that people who tried to diet more rigidly during weekends and holidays were actually at a higher risk of weight regain, not weight loss.[130]

### Self-Reported Diet Strictness from Successful Weight Loss Maintainers in the Portuguese Weight Control Registry[131]

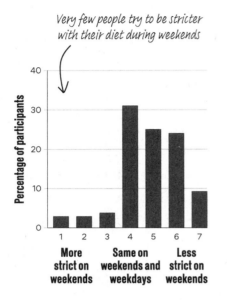

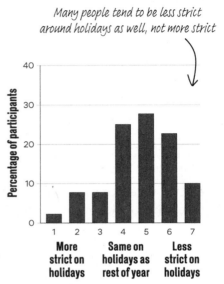

As it turns out, being consistently good can beat being sporadically perfect. So, if you are someone who is extraordinarily strict during the week only to find yourself going completely off the rails at the weekend, maintaining a more relaxed but regular eating schedule over the course of the week could help you develop a healthier habitual nutritional intake, which sounds like a smart idea.

If you would benefit from more consistency, here are some example starting habits for keeping a regular eating pattern:

- If you are someone who finds yourself with a sporadic eating schedule and this often triggers you to eat a lot more food at certain times of the day, it's obviously a sensible idea to try to resolve this. For example, you might play around and find out that you do well eating breakfast at around 9am, lunch at around 1pm and dinner at around 6pm with a couple of snacks in between, which then reduces your body's urge to scarf down huge catch-up meals in the evenings.

- If you are someone who diets strictly during the week and then all hell breaks loose between Friday and Sunday, you might do better relaxing your food rules during the week and shooting for more consistency. An 80 percent grade over the course of seven days beats a perfect 100 percent for four days and 20 percent on the remaining three days, you know?

- Likewise, if you are someone who tries to be incredibly strict all the time, including holidays, and this militant approach makes it difficult to stick to a healthy lifestyle for long periods of time without feeling like you are relapsing, relaxing it a little bit might make it less likely that you end up shooting yourself in the foot. Consistently good usually beats being sporadically perfect, so to speak.

## A Crucial Final Note on Habit Implementation

You know when you have a group of friends or a hot date coming over to your house, so you want to do a little last-minute cleaning to make sure the place looks nice and tidy before they arrive? Well, let's say you only have an hour to do the best job you can, what do you pick? You probably don't get a toothbrush and spend the whole hour cleaning the underside of the toilet or scrubbing the inside of the oven, do you? They can be very labor-intensive tasks that take a lot of work for not much visible payback. If you only have one hour to clean the place for other people, you have to pick the best-return-on-investment things to clean. Spending a few minutes vacuuming the floors, throwing away any visible trash and making sure you don't have dirty underwear on the floor will make your house look a lot cleaner for a lot less effort than spending an hour scrubbing the inside of the oven.

The idea behind this list of possible habits is for you to pick and choose things that suit your personal preferences to help take you from where you are now to wherever you want to be. But I would also like to make sure you don't waste energy focusing on stuff that doesn't matter much. Life is short, and the number of things you can choose to spend your energy on is finite, so please be selective with your choices. I spent a lot of my younger years obsessing over all the teeny-tiny health and fitness habits, tricks and hacks that I thought might get me from A to B faster, only to realize that most of them didn't even really move the needle, they just caused me a lot of unnecessary stress for almost zero payback. That is a terrible return on investment.

There is something called the Pareto principle, also known as the 80:20 rule, which states that 80 percent of outcomes come from 20 percent of causes. In the context of fat loss, health and overall well-being, a massive majority of your results can actually come from a surprisingly short list of behaviors. You don't have to pick all 13 of the habits in this chapter to work on, necessarily. I would be fucking delighted if all my clients focused on one or two of the following options: improving their sleep quality; consuming less alcohol; eating more nutrient-dense foods like fruits, vegetables, lean proteins, wholegrains and legumes; consuming fewer high-calorie, ultra-processed foods; exercising consistently or increasing their lifestyle activity levels.

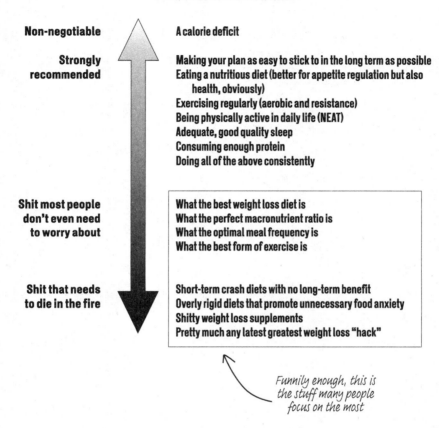

**Fat Loss Fundamentals**

**Non-negotiable** — A calorie deficit

**Strongly recommended** — Making your plan as easy to stick to in the long term as possible
Eating a nutritious diet (better for appetite regulation but also health, obviously)
Exercising regularly (aerobic and resistance)
Being physically active in daily life (NEAT)
Adequate, good quality sleep
Consuming enough protein
Doing all of the above consistently

**Shit most people don't even need to worry about** — What the best weight loss diet is
What the perfect macronutrient ratio is
What the optimal meal frequency is
What the best form of exercise is

**Shit that needs to die in the fire** — Short-term crash diets with no long-term benefit
Overly rigid diets that promote unnecessary food anxiety
Shitty weight loss supplements
Pretty much any latest greatest weight loss "hack"

*Funnily enough, this is the stuff many people focus on the most*

Now that you have some dietary strategies from Chapter 3 and some individual healthy habits from this chapter, let's move on to a topic that is woefully neglected in the health, fitness and weight loss industries: how you can become better at adhering to these in the long term and with less conscious effort.

# 6

# Skill-Building: Strengthening Your Habits

From a fat loss perspective, everyone already knows that what you eat and how much exercise you do are crucial factors for success, yet a shit-ton of adults globally struggle to stick to the plan they were excited by on day one.

If losing weight on a diet and exercise plan is easy, in theory, keeping that weight off in the long term should be equally easy. You know what habits and behaviors you implemented to lose the weight initially, so just keep doing them. That doesn't sound so hard, does it?

However, something that sounds very simple on paper can be extraordinarily difficult to implement. There is something called the "intention–behavior gap": you might know what behaviors you want to follow (the intention), but you struggle to put them into practice (the behavior).[1] In other words, intentions alone are not enough for behavior change to occur.

## The Intention-Behavior Gap

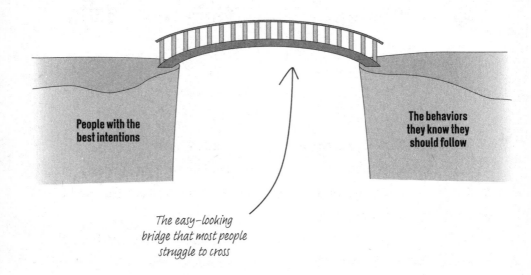

People with the best intentions

The behaviors they know they should follow

*The easy-looking bridge that most people struggle to cross*

Keeping weight off after the initial diet phase is actually so tricky for so many people that the National Institutes of Health in the US organized a team of experts to discuss what factors make long-term weight loss such an elusive creature and what can be done to help.[2] It isn't just about knowing what behaviors to follow, but understanding why adhering to them over a long period of time gets progressively harder. They discussed some of the things I have already talked about in this book, like genetics and appetite, and some things I don't plan on talking about, like weight loss drugs and surgeries. However, one novel thing they explored was the "overwhelming conclusion" that weight loss success needs to involve the expertise of behavioral researchers, rather than just focusing on physiology (like a lot of weight loss diets and weight loss books do). They agreed that weight regain was extremely common after six to nine months of a weight loss intervention and that, even at the point of maximal weight loss, a lot of the behaviors people embarked on have already started waning from an adherence perspective. It isn't that people don't know what to do to lose weight, the difficult part is actually overcoming the barriers that stop you doing those over a longer period of time. This is one of the reasons I have included a lot of self-evaluation in this book, because if you are aware of your own possible pitfalls, it gives you a much better chance of evading them and actually achieving successful long-term change.

From reading this book, you should hopefully have at least one goal written down. You should also have a list of individual healthy behaviors that you like the sound of to help you reach those goals. Now we are going to go one step further and discuss supporting skills that can help you bridge that intention–behavior gap that so many people struggle to hurdle with any real success. I like to view these as concepts that can strengthen and reinforce your ability to progress.

A review paper that looked at previous weight loss literature eloquently explains the need for this chapter:

> There is a large variability between individuals in the weight loss response to any given diet treatment, which fuels interest into personalized or precision nutrition. Although most efforts are directed toward identifying biological or metabolic factors, several behavioral and psychological factors can also be responsible for some of this interindividual variability.[3]

In short, a lot of you do not get the long-term weight loss results you expect, and while everyone is arguing about various nutritional approaches, like which diet plan is better than the others, there are likely some neglected underlying psychological influences that can help you toward, or hinder you from, achieving those results, so let's talk about some of them now.

## Behavioral and Psychological Factors That Can Influence Your Response to Diet and Lifestyle Interventions

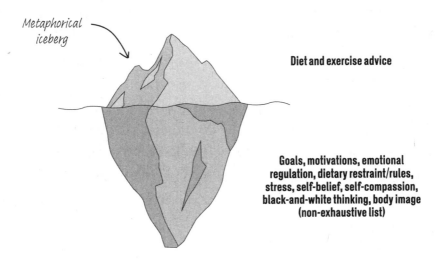

Metaphorical iceberg

Diet and exercise advice

Goals, motivations, emotional regulation, dietary restraint/rules, stress, self-belief, self-compassion, black-and-white thinking, body image (non-exhaustive list)

I am going to simplify the shit out of the following concepts for a couple of reasons. Firstly, they can be nerdy and boring, and if any of you really want nerdy and boring you can read the research papers I cite at the back of the book. Secondly, the research on them isn't as concrete as advice like "Reduce your calorie intake to lose weight" or "Eating vegetables is good for your health," which we have a hell of a lot of studies to support. Consider these as seeds I want to plant in your brain, if you think they apply to you.

## Emotional Regulation

This describes the ability to recognize when emotional responses are affecting your eating patterns, and reframing your thoughts to interrupt this pattern. Here is a direct quote from a research paper that interviewed people with obesity, to understand their own personal struggles:

> In Weight Watchers…it's like always speaking about the superficial…you can't go into a group of forty people and discuss and say "Well, I had an argument with my husband tonight, it's really put me off and I went into the fridge" or "I got fired from work" or anything like that. So those things you keep under cover, but the real reason you are not under control is because you are not approaching those issues and for that reason it never worked.[4]

If you have never heard or read anyone talking about the emotional side behind trying to lose weight, you might be mistaken for thinking this is a brand-new research paper where the information is yet to be popularized, but alas, this was actually published 20 years ago. Funnily enough, some of the biggest reasons that you might struggle to lose body fat and keep it off are actually things that most diet books discuss the least, if ever. People who regain weight after a dieting phase are often those who regulate their emotions with food,[5,6] and almost as worryingly, this information has been known for literally decades. For example, one research paper published way back in 1980 looked at some so-called "chronic dieters" who were able to lose weight repeatedly but not able to maintain that weight loss, losing and regaining nearly 40kg (over 80lb) each in 19 years of dieting, on average.[7] They found that unsuccessful dieters often reported stressful life events that made it difficult to manage their weight and binge eaters reported perfectionistic and rigid dieting attitudes that worked in the short term but were difficult to maintain in the long run (like we discussed in the previous chapter about prioritizing consistency—see page 174), hence the prevalence of yo-yo dieting. They also found that successful weight loss correlated with decreases in problem eating habits, causing the researchers to state: "Unlearning the behaviors leading to a relapse is just as important for such persons as learning techniques to promote weight loss."

Unfortunately, this isn't something that is easy to package up and sell, so chances are you won't have heard anyone talking about it in their fancy keto intermittent fasting revolutionary rapid weight loss extreme program. But what's the fucking point of people talking to you about calories and different diet plans without discussing the actual reasons you might want to eat more food in the first place? You aren't robots. You can't just have someone barking an order at you and you follow it with immaculate precision. You are humans, and humans are complicated little buggers.

Basically, a lot of diets and even weight loss clubs focus on the surface-level stuff without actually getting to some of the more important root problems, and if this is the first time you are reading about this idea, it shows how much the weight loss industry continues to neglect it. Nowadays, more scientific papers are acknowledging how emotional eating can impact weight gain and how important emotional regulation is when it comes to actually maintaining weight loss in the long term.[8] The most obvious example people probably think of is comfort eating when you are sad. Even in Hollywood films, you often see the kind of cliché example of someone breaking up with their boyfriend and then sitting on the couch and crying into a tub of ice cream. In the history of shitty life events, I have never seen someone bawling their eyes out deciding to self-soothe by biting into a cucumber or going out to a juice bar with their friends so they can drink a kale and ginger smoothie.

However, feeling sad or depressed are certainly not the only drivers of emotional eating; you might find yourself turning to high-calorie extra delicious foods when you are happy, bored, anxious, lonely, angry or stressed.[9] If you have a shit day at work and you feel your snack hand becoming increasingly fidgety, this applies to you.

Emotional eating is not a bad thing as such; it's natural for emotions to influence the way we behave, and the way we feel can sometimes change what we want to eat, much like how we often crave different foods depending on whether it's a hot summer's day or a cold winter's night, or whether you are out at a restaurant or snuggled up at home on the couch. A countless number of factors subconsciously influence what foods and how much of those foods you want to eat, including how you feel about your own body.[10]

There are a couple of different ways to approach this. Sometimes people who know they are emotional eaters will do things to interrupt or block this pattern, like choosing to exercise because they feel it puts them in a good mood, or talking to a friend if they eat more when they feel lonely, or not going grocery shopping when they are hungry or sad.[11,12]

The idea behind emotional regulation is similar to this, but you would interrupt the pattern by reframing your thoughts rather than trying to switch tasks. If you are someone who finds yourself nibbling between meals or overeating at meals when you feel stressed, finding strategies you could implement that would divert your focus could change this cycle.[13]

## A Hypothesized Model of the Impact of Food-Related Behaviors and Emotional Functioning on Body Weight in Adults[14]

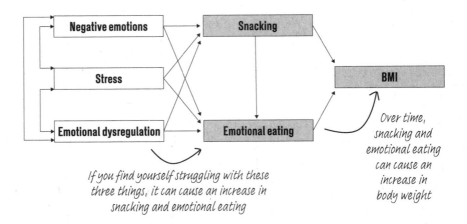

If you find yourself struggling with these three things, it can cause an increase in snacking and emotional eating

Over time, snacking and emotional eating can cause an increase in body weight

There are various psychology-based practices for treating emotional eating, including behavioral weight loss interventions, cognitive behavioral therapy, mindfulness-based treatments, and others.[15] While it is wildly outside the scope of this book for me to go into them in detail, one important thing that I would like to emphasize is something called cognitive reappraisal. This sounds like a semi-fancy term, but, in reality, it basically just means reframing something you are feeling, which can then change how you act upon it.

For example, I once tore my bicep off the bone in the gym, which I would describe as very suboptimal. I wouldn't recommend you try it. As someone who lifts weights a lot, I knew it would really fuck up my training and my brain started going into a spiral for how much this would screw up my life. Rather than doing what I used to do, and falling into a pit of depression, locking myself in my bedroom and stuffing my face with comfort food or using other harmful coping tactics, I reframed it.

Sure, it did stop me from doing any upper body exercise and did interfere with my work, but it also forced me into doing other forms of exercise that I had neglected, like doing more cycling, which was good for my health. By finding the silver lining on what seemed like a dark cloud, my brain was in a more positive space, and I kept up with an alternative exercise routine, which I was close to abandoning altogether (part of an all-or-nothing mindset, which we will discuss shortly).

Cognitive reappraisals can alter your attitude toward food,[16,17] which might be a useful skill to help support long-term weight management.[18,19] Not only that, but it can just be a very useful skill in general. As an example, here are three specific techniques that one research paper found increased participants' well-being, which have also been examined elsewhere:[20]

1. Positive reframing: Looking for the silver lining when a dark cloud appears. You feel like you have fallen off your diet. OK, what are the positives? How can you learn from your experience going forward?

2. Self-distancing: Step back from what you are experiencing and imagine you are someone else observing what you are going through. If you were a fly on the wall, watching yourself right now, what advice would you be able to give yourself? You are struggling to find time to go to the gym? OK, if you step back and look in on your situation, is there any advice or a solution you can give yourself?

3. Temporal distancing: Whatever you are struggling with right now, how would you feel about it later down the line? It might be super stressful in this moment, but will you give it much thought six months from now? If you are feeling pissed off that you ate a box of cookies, does future-you ten years from now actually give a fuck? Probably not. Nobody lies on their deathbed wishing they spent their adult life a couple of kilos or a few pounds lighter, you know?

Life does have a tendency to occasionally punch you in the face, and if you lie down in the corner of the ring every time this happens, you will probably find yourself hibernating there for eternity. Looking for silver linings and problem-solving your way out of adversity can be a very handy talent to have in all circumstances, not just something that could be beneficial for weight management.

## Cognitive Flexibility

This describes the ability to recognize that even the best-laid plans hit stumbling blocks sometimes. For instance, have you ever been on a diet and had a list of foods that you were never allowed to eat? Let's use cookies as an example. You spend a couple of weeks avoiding cookies like they are the plague, and things are going well, but then one day you succumb to temptation and inevitably nibble on a cookie. How do you feel? A lot of people who do this struggle to exercise cognitive flexibility. Instead, they have very intense feelings of guilt, like they have broken their dietary rulebook, and they suddenly think, "Fuck it, I have ruined my diet anyway!" and proceed to eat the rest of the packet, any other cookies they have in their pantry, plus the entire contents of their fridge. This is sometimes described as a "what the hell" effect and stems from the idea that eating a little bit of prohibited food somehow causes people to eat even more food as a result.[21] This can also be described as eating more food not because you are hungry, necessarily, but because of a "personal norm violation." You might feel disappointed, like you have let yourself down, even though you haven't objectively eaten a large amount of food.[22]

In the grand scheme of things, what negative impact does eating one single cookie have on your overall health? Absolutely fucking zero. If you are eating three nutritious meals per day, that's 1,095 nutritious meals per year. Even if you ate nothing but cookies for three entire days, that's still less than 1 percent of the year. Feeling terrible for eating one single cookie and then going on to binge eat because you feel guilty is like finding a nearly invisible scratch on your car and then getting so frustrated you decide to take a baseball bat to the rest of it.

As we touched on in Chapter 3, many people have a tendency to view things in black-and-white terms. Foods are either "good" or "bad," "healthy" or "unhealthy," "acceptable" or "prohibited," when, in reality, there is a vast spectrum of gray in the middle. Chocolate cake might not be the most nutritious food, and eating lots of cake every day obviously isn't a smart idea for your health, but that doesn't mean one slice is immediately going to ruin your diet. In fact, you could argue that being able to enjoy a slice of cake without guilt or shame actually enriches your life when compared with all the people who feel too anxious to even eat a single slice on their birthday.

This all-or-nothing thinking style is referred to as "dichotomous thinking"[23] and it's believed that people who have strong black-or-white views toward food may find it harder to maintain a healthy weight in the long term[24,25,26,27] and may be more susceptible to eating disorders.[28]

When I was a child, my mum always described me as a perfectionist. I remember being about 12 years old and spending hours on an art project where I had to paint a mountain. I loved painting and set very high standards for myself, and after I had worked on it for an unusually long time by adolescent homework standards, I didn't quite like what I saw. It was good, but it wasn't great. What did I do? I tore it up and threw it in the trash. Apparently, I would rather tell my teacher that I hadn't done the project than turn in something that didn't meet the very lofty standard I had set for myself, despite the fact I would get told off for not doing the work. This is how perfectionism can backfire—because perfectionists often give up on a task completely when they realize they can't complete it to the standard they hoped.[29] Instead of handing in a piece of work that was maybe 70 percent of what I wanted, I chose to hand in 0 percent and this made sense in my brain, for some strange reason.

In health and fitness terms, what could this look like?

- You have a list of foods you feel happy eating, and a list of foods you try to completely avoid at all costs, often feeling shame, guilt or disappointment for eating even a teeny-tiny portion of one of those foods.
- You refuse to work out unless you can complete your whole workout. If you normally train for an hour, but you only have a 30-minute window, maybe you view it as a waste of time and do nothing instead. Maybe you viewed the short "exercise snacks" section in the last chapter as completely worthless instead

of viewing it as a form of exercise that's better than doing nothing.

- You get stressed if you can't complete your workout plan exactly as it was written. If you normally use a piece of equipment in the gym that's broken, you want to just go home. If you are traveling and the local gym doesn't have what you want, you decide not to exercise at all.
- You try to follow an extremely strict and rigid dieting program, but then beat yourself up the moment you deviate even slightly from that unrealistic and overly optimistic plan.
- You view your lifestyle and diet choices as being "on" or "off"—just like someone who jumps on a diet plan in January, but jumps off again in February. In reality, health, fitness and well-being are just part of an ongoing life journey. It isn't like smoking, where people often say they are or aren't a smoker. What you eat and how much you move your body are constant dials that move up and down throughout your life, whether you pay them any deliberate attention or not.

Cognitive flexibility allows you to acknowledge and navigate these stumbling blocks to your best-laid plans. Life will occasionally throw obstacles at you, and sometimes these will hit you square on the nose. Just like you wouldn't completely quit your career if you had a couple of less productive days or weeks, there are going to be times when your health and fitness goals take a back seat to something else. But that's OK. Rather than insisting on being perfect or doing nothing at all, be adaptable enough to let yourself deviate from a strict path.

## Examples of Psychological Rigidity Compared to Psychological Flexibility

| Circumstance | Rigid Response | Flexible Response |
|---|---|---|
| You have less time to work out than originally planned | Skip your session entirely because you can't do exactly what you wanted to do | Do a modified, shorter workout because something is better than nothing |
| The piece of equipment you want to use is broken | Get pissed off and leave the gym because you can't follow the exact routine you wanted to | Do something else because, again, something is better than nothing |
| You ate an unplanned cookie | Think "Fuck it, I may as well eat the entire plate of cookies" and binge eat | Just enjoy the cookie (because cookies are delicious) and move on without guilt |
| You go out for dinner and the options are not foods you view as conducive to your diet | Think "These are bad foods I try to avoid completely" and get anxiety, or eat them and have a brain meltdown | Think "Sure, these are less nutritious, but they aren't 'bad,' they are just foods I should eat in moderation rather than abundance" |
| You made a big mistake on a work project and feel horrible | Stay in bed all weekend feeling sorry for yourself, skipping workouts and not eating well | Assess what happened and how to do better moving forward; shake it off and continue with your normal routine |

## Self-Compassion

Imagine that you have engaged in a "dietary lapse," which is a slightly fancy term for "Oh shit, I ate something that I do not think is conducive to my diet," like the cookie example I gave earlier. Rather than feeling guilty for breaking the rules of your diet, what would happen if you just…didn't feel guilty at all? What would happen if, instead of beating yourself up, you just enjoyed the cookie and moved on without hating yourself?

If this sounds like a radical idea, hold your horses for a moment. Needless to say, dietary lapses can risk the success of your overall diet.[30] If you start eating a shitload of high-calorie foods, this is obviously like shooting an arrow straight through any dieting balloon goal you might have floating around, and I am definitely not saying otherwise. However, let's probe this idea a bit.

Some research studies report that, on average, people who are dieting tend to have anything from three to twelve "dietary lapses" per week.[31,32] Now, that's a huge, barn-door-wide range, but one possible reason is that a "lapse" simply means an occasion during which you felt like you broke your dietary rules. If you ate an absolutely massive meal and then dived headfirst into eating five extra desserts because you only live once, you may view that as a lapse. But, if you were trying to avoid doughnuts and you ate one single solitary doughnut, then that could also be a lapse, despite it being much less significant in size.

There are two ways to improve your diet quality in this scenario:

1. Decrease the number of times that lapses happen.
2. Minimize the severity of the lapse.

The idea behind self-compassion links with what we discussed previously. Many people eat one cookie, feel guilty and then spiral into eating more cookies than they would normally. By cutting yourself some slack, it may interrupt that downward spiral cycle. One mistake many people make is thinking that being kind to yourself means you are less likely to hit your goal. But self-compassion isn't about complacency, more like acknowledging your mistakes and moving on, like a healthier response to an obstacle. Me throwing away my artwork as a kid because I didn't like it? That's zero self-compassion. Not being such an arsehole to myself, handing it in anyway, not being told off by my teacher because it actually looked like I did the homework, and learning from my mistakes next time I tried to do a painting? That would have shown more self-compassion and yielded a better result, not a worse one.

If your friend was going through a shitty period in life and beating themselves up, feeling like a failure, there is a strong chance you would support them through their pain, right? Well, why would you offer support to a friend but not to yourself? Self-compassion revolves around navigating three different but overlapping domains: self-kindness versus self-judgment, common humanity versus isolation, and mindfulness versus overidentification.[33]

1. Self-kindness versus self-judgment: Instead of condemning yourself for making a mistake, you offer yourself the same kind of encouragement you might be inclined to offer someone you love. This can decrease your feelings of unworthiness.

2. Common humanity versus isolation: If you fuck up, you might be inclined to think there is something wrong with you as a human and you are struggling with something other people find easy. In reality, you can feel less lonely in the knowledge that, with around 8 billion people on the planet, there is a strong chance that a huge number of people are going through a similar situation to you.

3. Mindfulness versus overidentification: If you are in pain or finding something difficult, acknowledging it can be an important step to understanding it rather than metaphorically sweeping it under the

rug and ignoring it. Being aware of and thinking about the issue sometimes runs away with us and we overidentify with that issue. You can fail at something, but that doesn't mean you are a failure as a human. Something terrible can happen in your life, but that doesn't mean that your whole life is terrible. Thoughts and feelings are transient, and they don't have to dictate the way you feel about yourself.

The science on self-compassion and weight loss is young and emerging, and, like a lot of psychological research, it is very far from concrete. Based on what we know so far, though, it could be very useful for weight loss as it can influence how you respond to so-called dietary lapses.[34] For example, one study did something mischievous to investigate this topic. They told the study participants that they wanted to test their experiences of eating in front of the television, so they gave them all one doughnut to eat.[35] What they were really testing was something a bit different. The doughnut was selected specifically because it was a "forbidden food" and, after the participants ate the doughnut, the researchers gave them a questionnaire to fill in and also gave them a bowl of candies for them to "taste test." The actual goal of the study was to see what happens when you decrease feelings of food guilt in some of the participants but not others, so after eating the doughnut, one group of the participants were told this by the researchers:

You might wonder why we picked doughnuts to use in the study. It's because people sometimes eat unhealthy, sweet foods while they watch TV. We thought it would be more like the "real world" to have people eat a dessert or junk food. But several people have told me that they feel bad about eating doughnuts in this study, so I hope you won't be hard on yourself. Everyone eats unhealthily sometimes, and everyone in this study eats this stuff, so I don't think there's any reason to feel really bad about it. This little amount of food doesn't really matter anyway. Just wait a second and I'll bring you the questionnaire.

Sure enough, the people who were told this by one of the researchers had lower levels of food guilt, and actually ate fewer candies afterward than those who didn't. While this was only one test study and the effects were fairly small, isn't it interesting that just 30 seconds of compassionate words from someone else is enough to change the way you feel about what you ate, and perhaps even cause you to eat less food as a result? Maybe feeling guilty every time you eat something you consider "prohibited" is doing you more harm than good?

Self-compassion may be beneficial for your body image and mental well-being as well.[36,37] If you are someone who has been struggling with your weight and you are also someone who has a tendency to bully yourself every time you feel like you have made a little mistake, perhaps self-bullying is part of the issue itself. Perhaps having more self-compassion would help you facilitate the healthy behaviors we discussed in the previous chapter. Even if it isn't from a weight loss perspective, life is too short to spend it treating yourself like shit.

## Your Important Take-Home Messages

On the surface, these skills don't sound like they are related to health and fitness at all, and you would be forgiven for thinking this is all far less exciting than a flashy sounding crash diet. However, these techniques can profoundly impact your ability to actually change behaviors in the long term. For example, telling someone to "stop binge eating" or "start exercising more" both sound like super-simple recommendations, but there is a vast chasm between how simple they seem on paper and how difficult they can be to actually put into practice. The supporting skills I've outlined in this chapter are the tools you need to build a bridge to cover that intention–behavior gap. You don't need yet another person telling you that exercise is healthy and a nutritious, reduced-calorie diet is paramount for weight loss. You need to dig beneath the surface and find out what you can do to make these easier for you to actually execute.

The most important take-home message from this chapter is that dieting in the short term is easy-peasy. You could randomly pick literally any terrible fad diet in the world and still lose a significant amount of weight over the next few weeks if you wanted to, not that I am suggesting that, obviously. But you can think of these a bit like get-rich-quick schemes. They all try their best to sound flashy and exciting, yet instinctively you know that, if it was that easy, everyone would be fucking doing it already.

However, these skills are a bit like secret character upgrades in your arsenal, or weapons that help you deal with obstacles and circumstances that you may have struggled to beat in the past. They aren't aggressive crash dieting tips; they are psychological skills that may not only make it easier for your long-term weight management, but can often enrich your life in other ways as well—and help you break free from that yo-yo dieting trap.

This is by no means the ultimate list of psychological factors that can impede or improve your ability to maintain your weight and well-being. For example, if you compare people who struggle with weight loss with those who are successful with it, there are some other things worth mentioning. Many people who give up on their journey do so because they are dissatisfied with the amount of weight they lose,[38] which is one reason why relying on the number on the scales as your primary motivational tool is not a smart idea. Having other more ingrained and autonomous forms of motivation, like exercising for enjoyment, can help you keep going even when weight loss slows down.[39] Because, as you already know, there are a bazillion fantastic reasons to exercise and eat a more nutritious diet that extend far beyond whether you lose weight or not. Learning from previous, often "failed," weight loss attempts so you don't keep making the same mistakes is always a good plan, as is trying to embed new behaviors into your daily routine, which you already know the importance of from Chapter 5.[40]

One of the most common reasons people often resort to overeating is because of the tendency to evaluate worth based on weight and shape.[41] Eating more because of how you feel about your own body is a difficult thought cycle to redirect, but doing so can assist with long-term weight loss.[42,43,44,45,46] This goes without saying, but you are not worth more or less as a human based on how you look or how much you weigh. I could not give a fuck whether you have a six-pack, how much you lift in the gym or what the number on the scales says when you stand on them; you aren't worth less than me or anyone else, and anyone who tells you otherwise deserves to be poked in the eye with a shitty stick.

Now that you have your baseline starting point, plus some dietary tips, healthy habits and supporting skills that you have chosen to implement as being beneficial for you, let's move on to the best ways to monitor your progress.

# 7

# Monitoring Your Progress

For a moment, imagine you are the owner of a big multimillion-dollar company. Recently, you have noticed that your profits are decreasing at a rapid rate, and you want to intervene before your whole company ends up in the toilet. So, you hire an expensive, very talented outside consultant to come in and look for the weak points and find the opportunities for growth. After doing an assessment, they write down an action plan for you and your team to help take you to new, uncharted territories—just like we have done in the previous chapters; the self-audit was the assessment of where your business is at now, and the habits were an itemized list of things your company can implement, and chances are there are a few things on that list that you did not realize before, but you know they make sense.

Now you have your personalized action plan, the consultant buggers off as you've spent the money to get their help and don't want to pay them forevermore. What do you do now to give your company the best chance of success? You monitor the changes and see how they correspond to your profits, expenses and any other data you care about, so you can tweak accordingly. If one avenue of your business really sucked, but you managed to turn it around, you know that the changes you implemented worked wonderfully, right? If another avenue was doing well but starts declining over time, you know that you need to fine-tune your approach to get it back on track.

This is the basic idea of monitoring your progress. It stems from a concept called "self-regulation," and the idea is very simple: if you monitor what you are doing, then you get feedback on whether it is working or not and this allows you to make appropriate adjustments—just like the business owner checking their sales figures and expenses.

## Why Is Self-Monitoring So Important? A Hypothetical Model

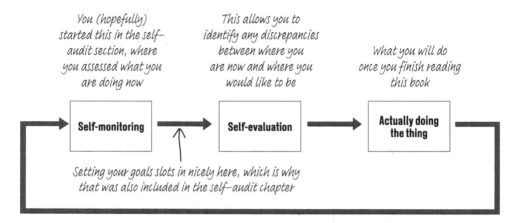

*You (hopefully) started this in the self-audit section, where you assessed what you are doing now*

*This allows you to identify any discrepancies between where you are now and where you would like to be*

*What you will do once you finish reading this book*

Self-monitoring → Self-evaluation → Actually doing the thing

*Setting your goals slots in nicely here, which is why that was also included in the self-audit chapter*

*This can be an ongoing process, where self-monitoring allows you to identify anything you want to change as you get closer to your goal, like a medical professional routinely checking health status*

Self-monitoring is so important that it has been used for decades, and has even been described as a "cornerstone" of weight loss treatment.[1] This shit is a big deal, to put it mildly. When it comes to health and fitness specifically, self-monitoring strategies tend to fall into three major groups: physical activity, diet and body composition.

## Your Physical Activity

When I was about 18 years old and relatively new to the gym, I remember someone telling me that I should log my workouts. They were a real smart cookie, but I didn't think their advice was necessary, so I ignored them. I exercised regularly and I was making progress, so I couldn't see the point of breaking out a notepad and writing down everything I did. To be honest, it sounded like a pain in the arse, and I couldn't think of much upside. I carried on resisting this advice when other smart cookies also told me to track my workouts until a couple of years later, when I finally caved in. Holy shitballs, Batman, I really missed the boat by not starting it sooner because I noticed things I hadn't even considered. By writing down what weights I lifted and for how many reps, it gave me a yardstick for what I wanted to beat next time. If I did 25 push-ups one workout, my goal in the next workout was to beat 25, and when I could see it written down in front of me, it gave me a big motivational kick up the arse in the best way possible. It didn't make me feel guilty if I failed, just excited to try to hit my goal.

It also had two other upsides. A few months later, I noticed I was hitting a lifting plateau. When I first started my new program, I noticed myself progressing very quickly, but now I was struggling to improve at all. Without my workout log, I wouldn't have been able to flick back through a couple of dozen pages to analyze that information, so it allowed me to psychologically draw a graph and realize that I wasn't going in the direction I had hoped, which encouraged me to change what I was doing.

However, when I flicked back a few more pages, what also slapped me in the face was just how far I had come. I was beating myself up for not making much progress on my last couple of workouts but, somehow, I had forgotten that six months earlier I couldn't even pick up some of the weights that I was now lifting comfortably for reps. That scruffy notebook with the ragged edges and the coffee stain not only helped me push harder in the gym, but it also kept me wanting to go back during a period when a lot of people would have given up completely. That shows how powerful self-monitoring can be.

A lot of the research on this aspect of exercise science is actually very basic. It's difficult to get 1,000 people to follow exactly the same weight-training program for a year, with half of them logging their workouts to see if they make faster progress than the other half who don't. It's much simpler to track something easy, like daily step count, as this can be measured with a simple pedometer you stick on your waist, or a smartphone or smartwatch that many of you have already. This is great news because it is also very affordable. If you were my client, I could buy you a cheap pedometer, give it to you and tell you to walk 10,000 steps per day, or tell you to walk 2,000 more steps than you do already (based on the information we could obtain in your self-audit), and just this advice alone could result in some weight loss and improvements to your health markers, like lowered blood pressure.[2] Or, you might already own a smartphone or smartwatch that could track your step count without you even realizing it, and people who use this function are often encouraged to walk more on a daily basis as well.[3] Tracking your step count can also be an especially good idea if you are dieting, because if you weigh less than you did before, your body may burn less energy from movement than it used to,[4] so walking more could help offset this. In fact, one research paper analyzed a group of people who were successfully maintaining a significant amount of weight loss and compared them to two control groups:[5]

1. A "normal weight" control group, who had a similar body mass index (BMI) to the successful dieters.
2. A "control with overweight/obesity" group, who had a similar BMI to the successful dieters prior to their weight loss.

It found that successful dieters walked far more than both control groups, which suggests that they rely on walking more as a tool to help them manage their body weight.

### Energy Burned via Physical Activity and Step Count Across Participant Groups[6]

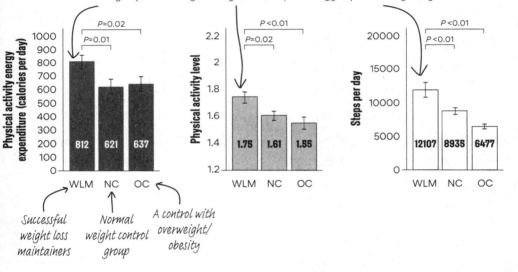

*Successful weight loss maintainers tend to walk more and burn more energy than the other groups, indicating this might be a useful strategy to prevent weight regain*

Technology is also advancing to better facilitate these habits using little psychological tricks. For example, some smartwatches have three physical activity rings on a digital display that fill up when you move, exercise and stand. If you hit your daily goals, the display does a little joyous dancy type thing to celebrate with you. As technology improves, there is a strong chance that it will incorporate more of these little psychological pats on the back to congratulate you when you move more, all with the idea of encouraging more physical activity.

Long story short, monitoring your physical activity can be a great tool to motivate you and help keep you accountable. It doesn't have to be complicated, and it absolutely should not add stress to your life. For example, if I spend all day working on my laptop, my smartwatch will nudge me to remind me that I have barely moved. I don't have to feel guilty about it, and sometimes it can be useful information to encourage me to take a break and walk around a little bit between tasks, just like one of the healthy habits that we discussed at the beginning of Chapter 5. If you want to get fancier, you can record your workouts in more detail; like how long you jog for and what distance you cover, or what weight-lifting exercises you performed for how many reps and sets. If you use it properly, it can help make exercise more rewarding, as it can help you hit little mini goals and track your progress in a way that most people do not bother doing. Seeing yourself getting fitter and stronger over time can help reinforce that the habits you are developing are working, and feeling like you are accomplishing shit on a regular basis is a nice psychological reward that can make you want to keep going.

## Your Diet

A client once came to me with the goals of losing fat and improving their health. They already went to the gym consistently, but weren't getting the results they had hoped for, so I asked them to keep a basic food and lifestyle diary for a week to see what we were dealing with. I always say to clients, "This is a judgment-free zone: if you spend your weekends binge drinking alcohol and taking an elaborate cocktail of class A drugs, it's better to tell me that than not tell me," because trying to make adjustments when you don't know the full story is a recipe for disaster. When the client came back, they showed me their food diary and a funny thing happened. They knew exactly what they needed to do without me even really having to open my mouth. The act of writing everything down can give you that extra clarity, and they realized that their overall diet quality was lower than what they wanted it to be. They were pretty sleep-deprived, consumed more alcohol than they thought, didn't really touch fruits and vegetables, and didn't consume much protein either. Those are four of the most important lifestyle boxes to put a metaphorical tick in, yet all four boxes were empty. Based on your own self-audit, there is a strong possibility that you noticed some things about yourself that you previously weren't aware of. For example, I have a pretty nutritious diet overall, but when I first wrote down what I ate daily, I suddenly realized that my consistency of eating at least five servings of fruits and vegetables was actually pretty shitty.

This is essentially how dietary self-monitoring began. In one study in the 1980s, people were given a notepad and asked to fill out a basic checklist of questions.[7] Rather than having the goal of losing weight and then trying to come up with ways to achieve that, they were encouraged to focus on smaller, individual behaviors, just like we have emphasized throughout this book. Let's use an example to show how much more effective this method can be. Imagine once again you have an identical twin, with identical weight loss goals:

Your twin's goal is to lose 10kg (22lb).
Your ultimate goal is also to lose 10kg (22lb), but instead of obsessing over that, your goal is just to consistently hit the healthy behaviors checklist you have drawn up based on the habits in Chapter 5.

Your twin goes to a weight loss group, and is applauded every time the scales go down and sometimes scolded when the scales don't move. Whether they feel success or shame entirely boils down to whether their body weight moves or not, which, when you think about it, sounds like a fucking terrible idea. You, on the other hand, have decided to do something different by just having a healthy habit checklist, like eating more fruits and vegetables, eating enough protein, and trying to get some decent quality sleep instead of doomscrolling on your phone at 2am. If I praise you for consistently adhering to healthy habits, it shifts the emphasis away from only caring about what the number on the scales says, which also decreases the likelihood of you feeling compelled to resort to unhealthy or even dangerous tactics to achieve those goals, like prolonged fasts, crash diets, saunas and laxatives.

Over time, dietary self-monitoring has evolved, and rather than just giving you a healthy habit checklist, you will sometimes be asked to fill in more detailed information like what you eat, at what time of the day and maybe the approximate number of calories in those meals.[8] Even when this is in super-simple notepad form, the people who record what they eat tend to lose significantly more weight than people who don't. Nowadays, notepads are viewed as prehistoric fossils that most of us never really bother with, because we have shiny gadgets like laptops, tablets and smartphones that allow us to make notes without carrying a pen and paper with us everywhere. So, if you want to record what you eat, you are probably going to do it on a website, or open an app on your smartphone, click a few times to select the food you ate, and it will help you estimate how many calories you are eating on a daily basis.[9] Although digital apps can vary wildly in terms of what fancy features they might be able to offer you,[10] they often show that they can help support weight loss goals compared to people not using the apps.[11] Basically, it doesn't necessarily matter whether you are using a notebook, a web app or a phone app, people who monitor what they eat tend to have more weight loss success than those who don't.[12] Technology can also be a great thing for other reasons, not just because it can help people who want to lose weight, but it can also make healthy advice more accessible. Not everyone can afford fancy customized diet plans with registered dietitians and tailored programs written by personal trainers, but digital apps can be a more affordable way to reach a wider group of people.[13]

This doesn't necessarily mean that everyone who wants to lose weight should start recording everything they eat, and there are definitely some dangerous traps that you don't want to fall into. For example, people who track their calorie intake can accidentally find themselves falling into a spiral of obsessiveness, trying to hit precise calorie intake goals every single day, which just isn't fucking realistic. Even if you followed the laborious task of weighing every single thing you ate and recording it down to the last calorie, you wouldn't ever know for sure how many calories you were really eating. For example, in America foods are allowed to be labeled with a 20 percent margin of error, so if a label tells you that your lunch food contains 500 calories, it may actually contain anything from 400 to 600 calories, and that is perfectly legal.[14] Even if you eat at a restaurant that has nutritional information on the menu, some of the meals might contain twice as many calories as what the restaurant tells you,[15] because it makes sense that a chef cooking things by hand is not going to serve exactly the same size portion of food thousands of times in a row when making the same dish, right? There is a concern that meticulous calorie counting could damage your relationship with food, and it has frequently been linked with eating disorders,[16,17,18,19] but some people appear to be able to track their calorie intake with no issues at all.[20,21]

Long story short, monitoring what you eat has been a common backbone of weight loss interventions for a long time, and it's arguably one of the most important things you could do to make sure you are eating in a way that is conducive to your goals.[22,23,24,25,26] But detailed calorie counting is viewed as such a burden for so many people that momentum is growing in the hunt to find simplified alternatives.[27] Several recent studies have tested various other ways that you can record what you are eating without having to be so meticulous.[28,29,30,31,32] That way, if the idea of weighing your food and recording everything you eat is about as appealing as repeatedly trapping your fingers in the door, or alternatively you start doing it and find yourself getting too obsessive, you can do something easier instead. After all, you aren't going to stick to something you hate doing, right? Some simplified examples include things like:

- only recording some foods that you eat, such as what you eat at weekends and holidays, plus weekday dinners
- only recording what you eat three or four days per week
- only recording "challenging" foods you want to eat less regularly, like candy, deep-fried foods, sugary sodas and restaurant dinners, which often tend to be surprisingly high in calories
- only recording "yellow" and "red" foods, basing this on the traffic light diet concept you see on the front of food packaging in some countries, where foods you are advised to eat less regularly are flagged red or amber and more nutritious foods are flagged green

## Example Habit Checklist Diary[33]

| The Habits | M | T | W | T | F | S | S | Done on 5 days or more? | Notes |
|---|---|---|---|---|---|---|---|---|---|
| 1. Prioritize nutritious lower-energy-density foods | ✓ | ✓ | ✓ | ✓ | ✓ | | | ✓ | This was easier for me to do during the week than the weekend. |
| 2. Eat more fruits and vegetables | | | | | | | | | |
| 3. Be mindful of extra dietary fat | ✓ | ✓ | ✓ | ✓ | ✓ | ✓ | ✓ | ✓ | I realized the creamy coffee I buy before work is higher in calories than I thought, so I swapped it for something that tastes just as nice. I have also decreased the amount of deep-fried food I eat. |
| 4. Prioritize lower-calorie drinks | | | | | | | | | |
| 5. Exercise more, at least to a point | | | | | | | | | |
| 6. Increase lifestyle activity | ✓ | | ✓ | | ✓ | | | | My job is still very sedentary, but I started walking with my partner on some evenings after work. |
| 7. Exercise snacks | | | | | | | | | |
| 8. Ensure adequate sleep quality | ✓ | ✓ | | ✓ | ✓ | | | | I realized when I play on my phone in bed it often takes me longer to get to sleep. I am working on improving this. |
| 9. Consume adequate protein | ✓ | ✓ | ✓ | ✓ | ✓ | ✓ | ✓ | ✓ | I noticed I didn't eat much protein at breakfast, only lunch and dinner. This was easy to change. |
| 10. Eat without distractions | | | | | | | | | |
| 11. Slow down when you eat | | | | | | | | | |
| 12. Engineer your immediate food environment | ✓ | ✓ | ✓ | ✓ | ✓ | | | ✓ | I started taking more nutritious snacks to work instead of relying on their vending machine. |
| 13. Keep a regular eating pattern | | | | | | | | | |
| Your weight | | | | | | | | | As I have a complicated history with the scales, I'm choosing not to track this at the moment. |

I am just going to say it: even people who enjoy tracking their calorie intake shouldn't want to do it forever. I can't imagine weighing food every day into my 80s because fuck, there have to be more enjoyable things to do with my time. This is why more research papers are exploring other options, like starting with more detailed self-monitoring and then transitioning to simpler versions—a bit like learning to ride your bike with training wheels before you remove them and go off alone.

If writing down what you eat and how much you exercise still sounds like torture to you, there is an even simpler option, which is more like a daily to-do checklist. Every work morning, I sit at my laptop and write down my tasks for the day, which gives me a teeny motivational goal-setting boost. I check off each task as I complete it and, over time, this not only helps make me become more accountable, but also builds my self-confidence when I see that I have the talent to finish what's on my list. I used to find to-do lists surprisingly daunting, but checking things off one by one slowly erodes those feelings of self-doubt I might have, which can help build momentum. On page 211 is an example of a habit-formation-based weight loss checklist, using the tips we talked about in the habits chapter, adapted for your reference.

*This diary template includes all 13 habits included in this book, but of course your own habit checklist may contain far less, or you can just focus on a few each week (see page 211 for an example). The idea is for you to use it as a template to suit your own personal preferences.*

# Habit Checklist Diary

| The Habits | M | T | W | T | F | S | S | Done on 5 days or more? | Notes |
|---|---|---|---|---|---|---|---|---|---|
| 1. Prioritize nutritious lower-energy-density foods | | | | | | | | | |
| 2. Eat more fruits and vegetables | | | | | | | | | |
| 3. Be mindful of extra dietary fat | | | | | | | | | |
| 4. Prioritize lower-calorie drinks | | | | | | | | | |
| 5. Exercise more, at least to a point | | | | | | | | | |
| 6. Increase lifestyle activity | | | | | | | | | |
| 7. Exercise snacks | | | | | | | | | |
| 8. Ensure adequate sleep quality | | | | | | | | | |
| 9. Consume adequate protein | | | | | | | | | |
| 10. Eat without distractions | | | | | | | | | |
| 11. Slow down when you eat | | | | | | | | | |
| 12. Engineer your immediate food environment | | | | | | | | | |
| 13. Keep a regular eating pattern | | | | | | | | | |
| Your weight | | | | | | | | | |

Of course, based on your own self-audit and what habits you selected in Chapter 5, you might want to change the contents of this table and there is no real reason you desperately need to start off with every habit. As discussed in Chapter 5, you might want to just start with one, two or three and, when you get good at completing those consistently, add another one, until you are where you want to be. Remember, if your goal is to improve your health for life, it makes sense to focus on long-term behavior change, so shoot for consistently building things into your routine until they become second nature, which will make it much easier for you later.

In the blank template on page 213, I would like to invite you to choose some habits that you think are suitable for you to start off with, and use this as the beginning of a daily habit checklist to get things moving, just ticking them off as you complete them. The goal here is to start building momentum, ingraining these habits into your daily routine so they slowly start to become second nature.

## Your Body Composition

If your goal is to lose weight, it makes sense that you need to periodically weigh yourself, right? It would be like having the goal of saving more money but never looking at your bank balance to see if your saving plan was working. I know it's pointing out the painfully obvious, but hopping on the scales is the best way of knowing how much you weigh. Nobody can disagree with the fact that the scales are the best tool for weight measurement because that's literally what they are designed to do. The real argument is around how important weighing yourself is to begin with and what you might want to do instead.

The scales do not tell you anything about your actual body composition. They cannot tell you how much muscle or fat tissue you have, or what percentage of your body is water. They simply put a number on your overall relationship with gravity. This causes issues because it often leaves people feeling happy every time the number goes down but distressed every time the number goes up, even when they have no way of knowing if the weight they've lost is body fat or not. You could gain 1kg (2.2lb) in less than 60 seconds, simply by drinking a liter of water. You will also gain weight every time you eat, and you might be surprised how many people get stressed when they realize they weigh a couple of pounds more than they expected, even though they weighed themselves immediately after eating. Many people weigh themselves not just once, but multiple times per day, despite the fact these short-term fluctuations are better at telling you what's happening to the contents of your stomach rather than whether you gained or lost body fat. Unfortunately, having your actual body composition tested is often difficult and expensive. None of you have expensive DEXA scan equipment sitting around at home, and those consumer-targeted electronic devices you stand on to predict your body fat percentage tend to be as accurate as a blindfolded monkey playing darts. Therefore, you are stuck with using the scales because they are cheap enough that you can have a pair at home. Basically, the scales aren't sophisticated enough to tell you much about yourself, and a lot of people have really fucked-up relationships with them, so, for some people, I strongly believe that an over-reliance on scales can be detrimental.

However, if you are aware of the possible pitfalls, weighing yourself regularly can still be a useful thing to do. If you go online and look at the New York Stock Exchange to find a huge company like Amazon, Apple or Microsoft and zoom in really closely, you will often see that the company share price valuations ping pong around all over the place. In a single week, they can move up or down multiple times, so if you were a newbie investor and wanted to gamble some money on what would happen in the next seven days, that could be a very risky play. But, if you zoom out to see what happens over several months or years, those daily fluctuations often level out and you can see the long-term trends. The daily jumps might not have told you much, but now you can see more easily whether a company has been growing or not over the past few years. This is essentially what weighing yourself can be like. Too many people obsess over whether they gained a couple of pounds overnight, or whether the temporary weight loss they saw when they got food poisoning and explosive diarrhea was a good thing or not (pro tip: it isn't), and I don't want you to fall into that trap. Instead, you might just want to see if your body weight is trending up or down over the course of several months, and normally this does correlate with whether you are losing body fat or not. If your body weight continually trends up, you know you are consuming more energy than you are burning, and this gives you a chance to change what you are doing, if you want.[34] If you don't ever step on the scales, you don't have this data to make an informed opinion.

If you want several decades of scientific studies summarized into a couple of short sentences, here you go. If your goal is to lose weight, weighing yourself regularly will probably help you with that goal versus burying your head in the sand and not weighing yourself at all.[35,36,37,38] In fact, if you look at people who lose weight successfully and keep it off for a long period of time, weighing themselves regularly is one of the most commonly reported behaviors.[39]

But everything has pros and cons, right? Therefore, it's crucially important that you are aware of the cons, too, so you can judge the risk-to-reward ratio for yourself. Standing on the scales regularly can mess with your emotions. One study found that weighing themselves frequently is a habit more commonly seen in people who suffer with an eating disorder and those who endorse disordered eating behaviors, and over a quarter of men and over half of the women surveyed reported that the scales also have the power to impact their mood.[40] This has been seen in other research papers, where women also reported that the scales not only had the power to impact their mood, but also their feelings of self-worth and how relaxed they felt about sex,[41] as well as making them feel more anxious and depressed, especially if the number was trending in the opposite direction to what they hoped for.[42] There is a lot more to your health than your body weight, and if something makes you feel like shit psychologically it's hard to consider that a wonderful thing, right?

In theory, outside of medical issues, which, of course, can make things more complicated, seeing your body weight go up consistently for a long period of time is a clear sign that any weight loss diet you are following is not working and it allows you to change what you are doing, which sounds like a great thing on paper. In reality, it often doesn't work like that. Many people who see they have gained weight actually disengage with their weight loss goal, rather than adapt what they are doing and keep going.[43] Giving up on a diet plan isn't always a bad thing, especially if that diet plan is overly restrictive dog shit that you hate following, but when people also stop exercising because they think it's not working, that becomes a major problem. If you have ever stood on the scales, didn't like the number you saw and thought to yourself, "Fuck this shit, it's not worth it anymore!," then you already know what I am talking about.

If you picked five healthy habits from Chapter 5, like exercising more, being more active in day-to-day life, consuming less alcohol, eating more fruits and vegetables, and improving your sleep quality, you could significantly improve your health, and lose body fat in the process (depending on how much food you are eating and how much exercise you are doing, of course), even if you never set foot on the scales again. This is why there is a growing trend for people to use a "weight-inclusive," "weight-neutral" or "health-centric" approach to their lifestyle, which basically means "Please stop worrying so bloody much about whether you lose weight or not and just focus on the individual behaviors that you know are healthy."[44,45,46]

## Why the Health-Centric Model Could Be a Smart Idea

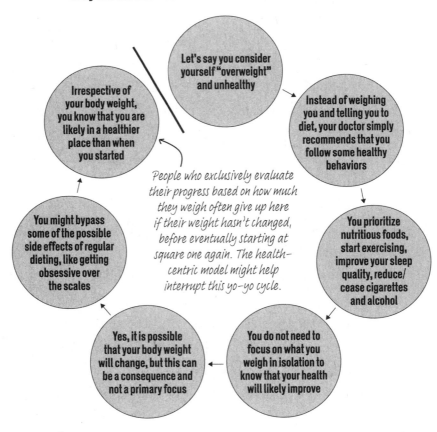

Let's say you consider yourself "overweight" and unhealthy

Instead of weighing you and telling you to diet, your doctor simply recommends that you follow some healthy behaviors

You prioritize nutritious foods, start exercising, improve your sleep quality, reduce/cease cigarettes and alcohol

You do not need to focus on what you weigh in isolation to know that your health will likely improve

Yes, it is possible that your body weight will change, but this can be a consequence and not a primary focus

You might bypass some of the possible side effects of regular dieting, like getting obsessive over the scales

Irrespective of your body weight, you know that you are likely in a healthier place than when you started

*People who exclusively evaluate their progress based on how much they weigh often give up here if their weight hasn't changed, before eventually starting at square one again. The health-centric model might help interrupt this yo-yo cycle.*

I would like to make one thing very clear: when I talk about risks, these are *possible* risks that might happen to some people, not *definite* things that will happen to all of you. Saying "Everyone should throw the scales in the trash" is a one-sided way of discussing a complicated topic. For example, although weighing yourself regularly can be a stressful experience for some of you, some research has shown that people who weigh themselves daily may have no negative feelings toward the scales at all[47] or can actually improve their relationship with the scales over time.[48] This is why it is never as straightforward as telling you all what you should do, but letting you weigh up the pros and cons and appreciating that you are all unique individuals with unique circumstances and preferences.[49,50]

You may want to "make peace with the scale" if you plan to use scales alongside your habit implementation. One study recommends weighing yourself daily and tracking it on a graph, without any pressure to lose or maintain weight, in order to see how your weight fluctuates daily and weekly. Once you have been recording your weight for a few weeks, you will notice a general range, usually a couple of pounds or kilograms in each direction. These changes might be down to water weight or change of routine, such as a holiday. Knowledge of this range then allows you to have a more positive relationship with daily weight fluctuations, making you more likely to continue using the scales over a longer period.[51]

Alternatively, if you are terrified of standing on the scales and don't feel like that is a safe and welcoming path for you to start venturing down, but you still want to have a kind of monitoring tool, there are other options that some people like. Back when I was in my early 20s, I fell severely ill with inflammatory bowel disease and lost nearly 23kg (around 50lb) in the space of just a few weeks. I went from being a fit and athletic personal trainer to being so frail I struggled to walk on my own, let alone exercise. I could barely eat anything, and I was going to the toilet two dozen times a day, so it's fair to say it was a pretty shitty situation, pardon the pun. When my health improved and I could start training again, I was desperate to get my healthier and more muscular physique back, and my sister told me I should take a photo of myself, for all the clients who hired me in a year or two and saw the fitness model body I might have managed to reobtain, but had no idea that I had ventured through the depths of hell to get there again. At the time, I was so embarrassed with how ill I looked that I didn't want to take a photo of myself even in private, but I have kicked myself for it ever since. Sometimes it's nice to see how far you have come, you know? It's not about hating how you look now and placing too much value on what you look like in the mirror. I actually strongly dislike the transformation photo culture where too much emphasis is placed on what you look like and less emphasis is placed on the things you can't see, like your overall well-being and how you feel. I also fear a lot of the transformation photo comparisons are fueled with at least a smidgen of shame and self-hatred, which I don't love the idea of. That being said, sometimes occasionally looking back at an old reference photo can show how you have changed health-wise as well. Just please don't do that obsessive thing of repeatedly comparing how you look now to a photo of how you used to look, or, even worse, a photo of someone else. While competitive bodybuilders and physique athletes who are judged exclusively on how they look often need to take lots of progress photos, this level of physique scrutiny can come with its own mental health ramifications, so I don't feel comfortable encouraging you all to do it.

You can also use clothing as a rough guide. If I work with a client who has absolutely no interest in weighing themselves, that's totally fine with me because I want them to be happy, of course. Sometimes they come into sessions and say things like, "I am not sure if I have lost any weight, but the trousers I wear to work are too loose for me now, so I had to buy a smaller pair" and this can be very motivating for them. Obviously, this doesn't really work with Spandex-infused super stretchy jeans or leggings, but a pair of non-stretch jeans will often let you know when you have lost body fat. Because your BMI (which only factors in your height and weight) cannot reliably estimate how much body fat you have, increasing numbers of people think that waist measurements are more important,[52] as they are better at predicting how much abdominal fat you have, which is a more reliable health risk factor than body weight alone.[53] If you are exactly the same height and weight as someone else, you will have exactly the same BMI, but if you have more muscle and a much smaller waist measurement, this probably indicates that you have less visceral fat, which is a good thing. Therefore, even something simple like whether you have to use different notches on your belt can sometimes be a crude indicator of whether you are losing or gaining body fat, and it doesn't require you to stand on the scales or get someone to wrap their arms around your stomach with a measuring tape.

Ultimately, self-monitoring is an often overlooked, yet very important common cornerstone of successful behavior change. By knowing the pros and cons of all the methods we have discussed in this chapter, you can pick any of them that appeal to you personally and try them out. Remember, you are allowed to change your approach in the future, so something might work really well for you now, but that doesn't mean you need to do it forever. The goal of this book is to arm you with the knowledge so you can make the best decisions for yourself moving forward.

# 8

# Where Do You Go from Here?

I have worked in the fitness industry for a couple of decades now and have had the pleasure and privilege of working with a diverse range of clients—from teenagers to older people, brand-new beginners to advanced athletes, people with shredded six-packs to people with high body fat percentages, non-disabled people to people with disabilities. Humans come in all shapes and sizes, and, statistically speaking, there is a strong chance that I have worked with someone who is a lot like you.

Out of all the people I have ever worked with, how many people do you think stuck with the plan in the long term but didn't notice any results? I will give you a hint: it is less than one and rhymes with the word "schmero."

I am extremely confident that anyone can get great results in the gym as long as three basic boxes are ticked. First, the plan you are following has to be good, obviously. You can work hard at something, but if the tools you are using are ineffective, it's a waste of your time. Many people pour their hearts and souls into starting a new business, but if their business plan is total shit then the business will never do well regardless of how hard they work. You can often get faster and greater results with less effort if you have a better plan. Second, you need to be consistent. You can have the best business strategy in the entire world, but if you spend your life getting drunk and partying instead of executing that strategy, that business plan is as worthless as a wooden frying pan. Third, I think it's a super smart idea to have realistic expectations. It isn't mandatory, because if you aim for the stars and fall short, you are still among the clouds, or whatever that wanky clichéd motivational quote says. However, I have seen too many people shoot for the stars, then get disheartened if they don't reach them in double quick time and decide to abandon their metaphorical space trip altogether. You can have the best plan and even execute it perfectly, but if you quit it completely in six months, you can't be surprised if you are still at square one a year later, you know?

As we've explored in earlier chapters, I think it is crucially important to understand that some people find losing body fat a lot harder than others. There are some lucky people who can maintain a visible six-pack year-round with minimal to zero effort, and there are some people who feel like they have spent their whole lives dieting and have consistently struggled to make any progress, despite putting in a shitload more effort than the naturally slim people. Anyone who denies this reality deserves a poke in the eye, because they truly cannot understand and empathize with those of you who feel exhausted from fighting what feels like a lifelong uphill battle. If losing body fat was easy for everyone, weight loss medications and surgeries just would not exist, yet they do, and those businesses are booming. There also wouldn't need to be a constant stream of fad diets and diet pills churned out on the conveyor belt of the multibillion-dollar weight loss industry, yet there are, and it continues to happen because many people are desperate and can't find the solutions they are looking for.

Part of the reason this is so vital to understand is because many of you who have struggled in the past often feel like something is wrong with your body, and if you aren't noticing progress then you might be wondering, what is the fucking point? But that often happens when the only important metrics for you are the number on the scales or what size jeans you are wearing. There is a hell of a lot more to health and fitness than that and, in my opinion, it's a shame that these yardsticks get a disproportionate amount of attention.

Even if you are someone who feels like you do everything right, but your fat loss is slow to non-existent, it shouldn't be the case that this feels like you are failing, because you're not. Looking after your health and well-being is a lifelong journey and you can choose to give it as much or as little attention as you wish because it is always there in the background, responding to the habits and behaviors you impose on it. All you need to do is pick one or two health-promoting behaviors to start with and, if you can implement them consistently, you *are* making progress, even if it doesn't always feel like it.

I can say with my hand on my heart that I believe all of you reading this have what it takes to get better results than you have been up until now. In fact, I am very confident with that prediction. Do you know why? Because you have read this book. You have shown to yourself that you are in a relatively small subset of humans who will willingly read a whole book about a topic that interests you. Nobody pointed a gun at your head. Nobody took your family hostage and made you read this as a form of ransom. You did it of your own accord, and that takes effort. If you can sit down and spend hours reading a book with 60,000-ish words, you know that you are the kind of person who has the dedication to chase a pursuit, you just need to make sure that it is a pursuit that interests you. Since you have read these chapters, which were stealthily packed with a lot of scientific rationale, you have shown you are not only a human with dedication, but you are also one armed with knowledge—and that's a potent combination for achieving great things, if you want. You have the power to decide how you want to put this knowledge into action.

Once again, for a final moment, I would like to pretend you are my client and I am your trainer. When you picked up this book and started reading, you metaphorically hired me and I am emotionally invested in trying to help you get to a better place, wherever that may be. I genuinely care about your progress, so, as we depart this book journey together, I just want to leave you with some final words.

Every single one of you who started reading this book did so because you have an interest in losing body fat. Some of you might just be reading it from an educational perspective, or maybe because you follow me on social media and you want to support me, but chances are a majority of you are proactively dieting yourselves. Even if your only goal when you picked up this book was to lose body fat, I would like to remind you that how much you weigh and how much body fat you have are physical characteristics, a bit like your eye color or what hairstyle you have. Sure, they can have an impact on your health, but they are by no means the only things that can do this.

Although this book looks like it is about fat loss as a focused topic, it actually isn't. It is my attempt at bringing all of you who have been dieting into a room and then trying my best to funnel you toward a healthier, and more sustainable, path, whatever that looks like for you. Too many people obsess over trying to achieve their dream body and then spiral down a road that turns into a nightmare. If you follow a diet only to inadvertently sacrifice your overall health and well-being, then I wouldn't view that diet as successful, regardless of what the number on the scales says.

You are, always have been and always will be a worthy human, and how much you weigh is one of the least interesting things about you. Please don't be one of those people who give up 95 percent of their happiness just to weigh 5 percent less. Life is far too short and too precious to spend it hating yourself and feeling miserable. If you use the information in this book to become a healthier and happier human one year from now, I have achieved the goal I set out to when I first started writing.

## Things People Focus On

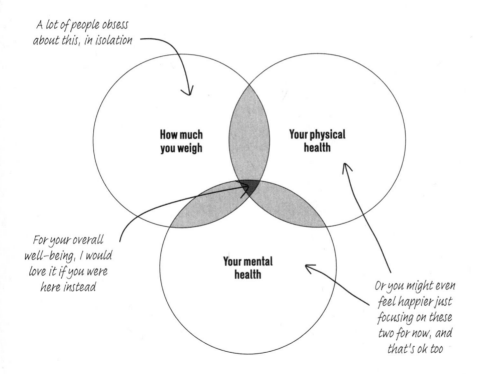

A lot of people obsess about this, in isolation

How much you weigh

Your physical health

Your mental health

For your overall well-being, I would love it if you were here instead

Or you might even feel happier just focusing on these two for now, and that's ok too

# References

## Introduction

1. Gjestvang, C., Abrahamsen, F., Stensrud, T., & Haakstad, L. A. H. (2020). Motives and Barriers to Initiation and Sustained Exercise Adherence in a Fitness Club Setting—A One-Year Follow-Up Study. *Scandinavian Journal of Medicine & Science in Sports*, 30(9), 1796–1805. https://doi.org/10.1111/sms.13736

2. Sperandei, S., Vieira, M. C., & Reis, A. C. (2016). Adherence to Physical Activity in an Unsupervised Setting: Explanatory Variables for High Attrition Rates Among Fitness Center Members. *Journal of Science and Medicine in Sport*, 19(11), 916–20. https://doi.org/10.1016/j.jsams.2015.12.522

3. Martin, C. B., Herrick, K. A., Sarafrazi, N., & Ogden, C. L. (2018). Attempts to Lose Weight Among Adults in the United States, 2013–2016. *NCHS Data Brief*, (313), 1–8.

4. Santos, I., Sniehotta, F. F., Marques, M. M., Carraça, E. V., & Teixeira, P. J. (2017). Prevalence of Personal Weight Control Attempts in Adults: A Systematic Review and Meta-Analysis. *Obesity Reviews: An Official Journal of the International Association for the Study of Obesity*, 18(1), 32–50. https://doi.org/10.1111/obr.12466

5. Haakstad, L. A. H., Stensrud, T., Rugseth, G., & Gjestvang, C. (2022). Weight Cycling and Dieting Behavior in Fitness Club Members. *Frontiers in Endocrinology*, 13, 851887. https://doi.org/10.3389/fendo.2022.851887

## Chapter 1

1. Baillot, A., Chenail, S., Barros Polita, N., Simoneau, M., Libourel, M., Nazon, E., Riesco, E., Bond, D. S., & Romain, A. J. (2021). Physical Activity Motives, Barriers, and Preferences in People With Obesity: A Systematic Review. *PloS One*, 16(6), e0253114. https://doi.org/10.1371/journal.pone.0253114

2. Ibid.

3. Poulimeneas, D., Anastasiou, C. A., Kokkinos, A., Panagiotakos, D. B., & Yannakoulia, M. (2021). Motives for Weight Loss and Weight Loss Maintenance: Results From the MedWeight Study. *Journal of Human Nutrition and Dietetics: The Official Journal of the British Dietetic Association*, 34(3), 504–10. https://doi.org/10.1111/jhn.12856

4. Major, B., Rathbone, J. A., Blodorn, A., & Hunger, J. M. (2020). The Countervailing Effects of Weight Stigma on Weight Loss Motivation and Perceived Capacity for Weight Control. *Personality & Social Psychology*

*Bulletin*, 46(9), 1331–43. https://doi.org/10.1177/0146167220903184

5. NCD Risk Factor Collaboration (NCD-RisC) (2017). Worldwide Trends in Body-Mass Index, Underweight, Overweight, and Obesity From 1975 to 2016: A Pooled Analysis of 2416 Population-Based Measurement Studies in 128.9 Million Children, Adolescents, and Adults. *The Lancet*, 390(10113), 2627–42. https://doi.org/10.1016/S0140-6736(17)32129-3

6. Kim, M. S., Kim, W. J., Khera, A. V., Kim, J. Y., Yon, D. K., Lee, S. W., Shin, J. I., & Won, H. H. (2021). Association Between Adiposity and Cardiovascular Outcomes: An Umbrella Review and Meta-Analysis of Observational and Mendelian Randomization Studies. *European Heart Journal*, 42(34), 3388–403. https://doi.org/10.1093/eurheartj/ehab454

7. Benn, M., Marott, S. C. W., Tybjærg-Hansen, A., & Nordestgaard, B. G. (2023). Obesity Increases Heart Failure Incidence and Mortality: Observational and Mendelian Randomization Studies Totalling Over 1 Million Individuals. *Cardiovascular Research*, 118(18), 3576–85. https://doi.org/10.1093/cvr/cvab368

8. Kyrgiou, M., Kalliala, I., Markozannes, G., Gunter, M. J., Paraskevaidis, E., Gabra, H., Martin-Hirsch, P., & Tsilidis, K. K. (2017). Adiposity and Cancer at Major Anatomical Sites: Umbrella Review of the Literature. *BMJ*, 356, j477. https://doi.org/10.1136/bmj.j477

9. Jayedi, A., Soltani, S., Motlagh, S. Z., Emadi, A., Shahinfar, H., Moosavi, H., & Shab-Bidar, S. (2022). Anthropometric and Adiposity Indicators and Risk of Type 2 Diabetes: Systematic Review and Dose-Response Meta-Analysis of Cohort Studies. *BMJ*, 376, e067516. https://doi.org/10.1136/bmj-2021-067516

10. Zheng, H., & Chen, C. (2015). Body Mass Index and Risk of Knee Osteoarthritis: Systematic Review and Meta-Analysis of Prospective Studies. *BMJ Open*, 5(12), e007568. https://doi.org/10.1136/bmjopen-2014-007568

11. Ul-Haq, Z., Mackay, D. F., Fenwick, E., & Pell, J. P. (2013). Meta-Analysis of the Association Between Body Mass Index and Health-Related Quality of Life Among Adults, Assessed by the SF-36. *Obesity*, 21(3), E322–7. https://doi.org/10.1002/oby.20107

12. Global BMI Mortality Collaboration, Di Angelantonio, E., Bhupathiraju, ShN., Wormser, D., Gao, P., Kaptoge, S., Berrington de Gonzalez, A., Cairns, B. J., Huxley, R., Jackson, C. L., Joshy, G., Lewington, S., Manson, J. E., Murphy, N., Patel, A. V., Samet, J. M., Woodward, M., Zheng, W., Zhou, M., Bansal, N.,...Hu, F. B.

(2016). Body-Mass Index and All-Cause Mortality: Individual-Participant-Data Meta-Analysis of 239 Prospective Studies in Four Continents. *The Lancet*, 388(10046), 776–86. https://doi.org/10.1016/S0140-6736(16)30175-1

13. Dwyer, J. T., & Mayer, J. (1970). Potential Dieters: Who Are They? *Journal of the American Dietetic Association*, 56(6), 510–14. https://doi.org/10.1016/S0002-8223(21)13354-1

14. Williamson, D. F., Serdula, M. K., Anda, R. F., Levy, A., & Byers, T. (1992). Weight Loss Attempts in Adults: Goals, Duration, and Rate of Weight Loss. *American Journal of Public Health*, 82(9), 1251–7. https://doi.org/10.2105/ajph.82.9.1251

15. Serdula, M. K., Williamson, D. F., Anda, R. F., Levy, A., Heaton, A., & Byers, T. (1994). Weight Control Practices in Adults: Results of a Multistate Telephone Survey. *American Journal of Public Health*, 84(11), 1821–4. https://doi.org/10.2105/ajph.84.11.1821

16. Han, L., You, D., Zeng, F., Feng, X., Astell-Burt, T., Duan, S., & Qi, L. (2019). Trends in Self-Perceived Weight Status, Weight Loss Attempts, and Weight Loss Strategies Among Adults in the United States, 1999–2016. *JAMA Network Open*, 2(11), e1915219. https://doi.org/10.1001/jamanetworkopen.2019.15219

17. Martin, C. B., et al. Attempts to Lose Weight Among Adults in the United States, 2013–2016. *NCHS Data Brief*.

18. McDow, K. B., Nguyen, D. T., Herrick, K. A., & Akinbami, L. J. (2019). Attempts to Lose Weight Among Adolescents Aged 16–19 in the United States, 2013–2016. *NCHS Data Brief*, (340), 1–8.

19. NCD Risk Factor Collaboration (NCD-RisC). Worldwide Trends in Body-Mass Index, Underweight, Overweight, and Obesity From 1975 to 2016.

20. Malik, V. S., Willett, W. C., & Hu, F. B. (2013). Global Obesity: Trends, Risk Factors and Policy Implications. *Nature Reviews: Endocrinology*, 9(1), 13–27. https://doi.org/10.1038/nrendo.2012.199

21. Hall, K. D. (2018). Did the Food Environment Cause the Obesity Epidemic? *Obesity*, 26(1), 11–13. https://doi.org/10.1002/oby.22073

22. McAllister, E. J., Dhurandhar, N. V., Keith, S. W., Aronne, L. J., Barger, J., Baskin, M., Benca, R. M., Biggio, J., Boggiano, M. M., Eisenmann, J. C., Elobeid, M., Fontaine, K. R., Gluckman, P., Hanlon, E. C., Katzmarzyk, P., Pietrobelli, A., Redden, D. T., Ruden, D. M., Wang, C., Waterland, R. A.,…Allison, D. B. (2009). Ten Putative Contributors to the Obesity Epidemic. *Critical Reviews in Food Science and Nutrition*, 49(10), 868–913. https://doi.org/10.1080/10408390903372599

23. Ross, S. E., Flynn, J. I., & Pate, R. R. (2016). What Is Really Causing the Obesity Epidemic? A Review of Reviews in Children and Adults. *Journal of Sports Sciences*, 34(12), 1148–53. https://doi.org/10.1080/02640414.2015.1093650

24. Villablanca, P. A., Alegria, J. R., Mookadam, F., Holmes, D. R., Jr., Wright, R. S., & Levine, J. A. (2015). Nonexercise Activity Thermogenesis in Obesity Management. *Mayo Clinic Proceedings*, 90(4), 509–19. https://doi.org/10.1016/j.mayocp.2015.02.001

25. Rizzato, A., Marcolin, G., & Paoli, A. (2022). Non-exercise Activity Thermogenesis in the Workplace: The Office Is on Fire. *Frontiers in Public Health*, 10, 1024856. https://doi.org/10.3389/fpubh.2022.1024856

26. Levine, J. A., Vander Weg, M. W., Hill, J. O., & Klesges, R. C. (2006). Non-exercise Activity Thermogenesis: The Crouching Tiger Hidden Dragon of Societal Weight Gain. *Arteriosclerosis, Thrombosis, and Vascular Biology*, 26(4), 729–36. https://doi.org/10.1161/01.ATV.0000205848.83210.73

27. Church, T. S., Thomas, D. M., Tudor-Locke, C., Katzmarzyk, P. T., Earnest, C. P., Rodarte, R. Q., Martin, C. K., Blair, S. N., & Bouchard, C. (2011). Trends Over 5 Decades in US Occupation-Related Physical Activity and Their Associations With Obesity. *PloS One*, 6(5), e19657. https://doi.org/10.1371/journal.pone.0019657

28. McDonald's (n.d.). Franchising Overview. Retrieved from https://corporate.mcdonalds.com/corpmcd/franchising-overview.html

29. KFC (n.d.). Our Locations. Retrieved from https://global.kfc.com/our-locations

30. Yum! (n.d.). Pizza Hut. No One Outpizzas the Hut. Retrieved from https://www.yum.com/wps/portal/yumbrands/Yumbrands/company/our-brands/pizza-hut

31. Restaurant Brands International (n.d.). Brands. Retrieved from https://www.rbi.com/English/brands

32. Guthrie, J. F., Lin, B. H., & Frazao, E. (2002). Role of Food Prepared Away From Home in the American Diet, 1977–78 Versus 1994–96: Changes and Consequences. *Journal of Nutrition Education and Behavior*, 34(3), 140–50. https://doi.org/10.1016/s1499-4046(06)60083-3

33. McCrory, M. A., Harbaugh, A. G., Appeadu, S., & Roberts, S. B. (2019). Fast-Food Offerings in the United States in 1986, 1991, and 2016 Show Large Increases in Food Variety, Portion Size, Dietary Energy, and Selected Micronutrients. *Journal of the Academy of Nutrition and Dietetics*, 119(6), 923–33. https://doi.org/10.1016/j.jand.2018.12.004

34. Young, L. R., & Nestle, M. (2002). The Contribution of Expanding Portion Sizes to the US Obesity Epidemic. *American Journal of Public Health*, 92(2), 246–9. https://doi.org/10.2105/ajph.92.2.246

35. Young, L. R., & Nestle, M. (2021). Portion Sizes of Ultra-Processed Foods in the United States, 2002 to 2021. *American Journal of Public Health*, 111(12), 2223–6. https://doi.org/10.2105/AJPH.2021.306513

36. Ibid.

37. Hoy, M. K., Clemens, J. C., Murayi, T., & Moshfegh, A. (2022). Restaurant Food Consumption by US Adults: What We Eat in America, NHANES 2017–2018. In: *FSRG Dietary Data Briefs*. United States Department of Agriculture (USDA).

38. Fraser, L. K., Edwards, K. L., Cade, J., & Clarke, G. P. (2010). The Geography of Fast Food Outlets: A Review. *International Journal of Environmental Research and Public Health*, 7(5), 2290–308. https://doi.org/10.3390/ijerph7052290

39. Hasan, H., Faris, M. A. E., Mohamad, M. N., Al Dhaheri, A. S., Hashim, M., Stojanovska, L., Al Daour, R., Rashid, M., El-Farra, L., Alsuwaidi, A., Altawfiq, H., Erwa, Z., & Cheikh Ismail, L. (2021). Consumption, Attitudes, and Trends of Vending Machine Foods at a University Campus: A Cross-Sectional Study. *Foods*, 10(9), 2122. https://doi.org/10.3390/foods10092122

40. Cooke, C. B., Greatwood, H. C., McCullough, D., Kirwan, R., Duckworth, L. C., Sutton, L., & Gately, P. J. (2024). The Effect of Discretionary Snack Consumption on Overall Energy Intake, Weight Status, and Diet Quality: A Systematic Review. *Obesity Reviews: An Official Journal of the International Association for the Study of Obesity*, 25(4), e13693. https://doi.org/10.1111/obr.13693

41. Centers for Disease Control and Prevention (2018). Characteristics of Vending Machines Available to Students in US Schools: Results from the School Health Policies and Practices Study, 2014. Atlanta, GA: US Department of Health and Human Services.

42. Neumark-Sztainer, D., French, S. A., Hannan, P. J., Story, M., & Fulkerson, J. A. (2005). School Lunch and Snacking Patterns Among High School Students: Associations With School Food Environment and Policies. *The International Journal of Behavioral Nutrition and Physical Activity*, 2(1), 14. https://doi.org/10.1186/1479-5868-2-14

43. Rovner, A. J., Nansel, T. R., Wang, J., & Iannotti, R. J. (2011). Food Sold in School Vending Machines Is Associated With Overall Student Dietary Intake. *The Journal of Adolescent Health: Official Publication of the Society for Adolescent Medicine*, 48(1),

13–19. https://doi.org/10.1016/j.jadohealth.2010.08.021

44. Pasch, K. E., Lytle, L. A., Samuelson, A. C., Farbakhsh, K., Kubik, M. Y., & Patnode, C. D. (2011). Are School Vending Machines Loaded With Calories and Fat: An Assessment of 106 Middle and High Schools. *The Journal of School Health*, 81(4), 212–18. https://doi.org/10.1111/j.1746–1561.2010.00581.x

45. Whatnall, M. C., Patterson, A. J., & Hutchesson, M. J. (2020). Effectiveness of Nutrition Interventions in Vending Machines to Encourage the Purchase and Consumption of Healthier Food and Drinks in the University Setting: A Systematic Review. *Nutrients*, 12(3), 876. https://doi.org/10.3390/nu12030876

46. Lawrence, S., Boyle, M., Craypo, L., & Samuels, S. (2009). The Food and Beverage Vending Environment in Health Care Facilities Participating in the Healthy Eating, Active Communities Program. *Pediatrics*, 123 Suppl 5, S287–92. https://doi.org/10.1542/peds.2008-2780G

47. Bell, C., Pond, N., Davies, L., Francis, J. L., Campbell, E., & Wiggers, J. (2013). Healthier Choices in an Australian Health Service: A Pre-post Audit of an Intervention to Improve the Nutritional Value of Foods and Drinks in Vending Machines and Food Outlets. *BMC Health Services Research*, 13, 492. https://doi.org/10.1186/1472-6963-13-492

48. Pechey, R., Jenkins, H., Cartwright, E., & Marteau, T. M. (2019). Altering the Availability of Healthier vs. Less Healthy Items in UK Hospital Vending Machines: A Multiple Treatment Reversal Design. *The International Journal of Behavioral Nutrition and Physical Activity*, 16(1), 114. https://doi.org/10.1186/s12966-019-0883-5

49. Kelly, B., Flood, V. M., Bicego, C., & Yeatman, H. (2012). Derailing Healthy Choices: An Audit of Vending Machines at Train Stations in NSW. *Health Promotion Journal of Australia: Official Journal of Australian Association of Health Promotion Professionals*, 23(1), 73–5. https://doi.org/10.1071/he12073

50. Thorndike, A. N., Sonnenberg, L., Riis, J., Barraclough, S., & Levy, D. E. (2012). A 2-Phase Labeling and Choice Architecture Intervention to Improve Healthy Food and Beverage Choices. *American Journal of Public Health*, 102(3), 527–33. https://doi.org/10.2105/AJPH.2011.300391

51. LaFata, E. M., Allison, K. C., Audrain-McGovern, J., & Forman, E. M. (2024). Ultra-Processed Food Addiction: A Research Update. *Current Obesity Reports*, 13(2), 214–23. https://doi.org/10.1007/s13679-024-00569-w

52. Van Boekel, M., Fogliano, V., Pellegrini, N., Stanton, C., Scholz, G., Lalljie, S., Somoza, V., Knorr, D., Jasti, P. R., & Eisenbrand, G. (2010). A Review on the Beneficial Aspects of Food Processing. *Molecular Nutrition & Food Research*, 54(9), 1215–47. https://doi.org/10.1002/mnfr.200900608

53. Weaver, C. M., Dwyer, J., Fulgoni, V. L., III, King, J. C., Leveille, G. A., MacDonald, R. S., Ordovas, J., & Schnakenberg, D. (2014). Processed Foods: Contributions to Nutrition. *The American Journal of Clinical Nutrition*, 99(6), 1525–42. https://doi.org/10.3945/ajcn.114.089284

54. Price, E. J., Du, M., McKeown, N. M., Batterham, M. J., & Beck, E. J. (2024). Excluding Whole Grain-Containing Foods From the NOVA Ultraprocessed Food Category: A Cross-Sectional Analysis of the Impact on Associations With Cardiometabolic Risk Measures. *The American Journal of Clinical Nutrition*, 119(5), 1133–42. https://doi.org/10.1016/j.ajcnut.2024.02.017

55. Chen, Z., Khandpur, N., Desjardins, C., Wang, L., Monteiro, C. A., Rossato, S. L., Fung, T. T., Manson, J. E., Willett, W. C., Rimm, E. B., Hu, F. B., Sun, Q., & Drouin-Chartier, J. P. (2023). Ultra-Processed Food Consumption and Risk of Type 2 Diabetes: Three Large Prospective US Cohort Studies. *Diabetes Care*, 46(7), 1335–44. https://doi.org/10.2337/dc22-1993

56. Wang, L., Du, M., Wang, K., Khandpur, N., Rossato, S. L., Drouin-Chartier, J. P., Steele, E. M., Giovannucci, E., Song, M., & Zhang, F. F. (2022). Association of Ultra-Processed Food Consumption With Colorectal Cancer Risk Among Men and Women: Results From Three Prospective US Cohort Studies. *BMJ*, 378, e068921. https://doi.org/10.1136/bmj-2021-068921

57. Lane, M. M., Gamage, E., Du, S., Ashtree, D. N., McGuinness, A. J., Gauci, S., Baker, P., Lawrence, M., Rebholz, C. M., Srour, B., Touvier, M., Jacka, F. N., O'Neil, A., Segasby, T., & Marx, W. (2024). Ultra-Processed Food Exposure and Adverse Health Outcomes: Umbrella Review of Epidemiological Meta-Analyses. *BMJ*, 384, e077310. https://doi.org/10.1136/bmj-2023-077310

58. Hall, K. D., Ayuketah, A., Brychta, R., Cai, H., Cassimatis, T., Chen, K. Y., Chung, S. T., Costa, E., Courville, A., Darcey, V., Fletcher, L. A., Forde, C. G., Gharib, A. M., Guo, J., Howard, R., Joseph, P. V., McGehee, S., Ouwerkerk, R., Raisinger, K., Rozga, I.,...Zhou, M. (2019). Ultra-Processed Diets Cause Excess Calorie Intake and Weight Gain: An Inpatient Randomized Controlled Trial

of Ad Libitum Food Intake. *Cell Metabolism*, 30(1), 67–77.e3. https://doi.org/10.1016/j.cmet.2019.05.008

59. Ibid.

60. Russell, S. J., Croker, H., & Viner, R. M. (2019). The Effect of Screen Advertising on Children's Dietary Intake: A Systematic Review and Meta-Analysis. *Obesity Reviews: An Official Journal of the International Association for the Study of Obesity*, 20(4), 554–68. https://doi.org/10.1111/obr.12812

61. Coleman, P. C., Hanson, P., Van Rens, T., & Oyebode, O. (2022). A Rapid Review of the Evidence for Children's TV and Online Advertisement Restrictions to Fight Obesity. *Preventive Medicine Reports*, 26, 101717. https://doi.org/10.1016/j.pmedr.2022.101717

62. Juul, F., Parekh, N., Martinez-Steele, E., Monteiro, C. A., & Chang, V. W. (2022). Ultra-Processed Food Consumption Among US Adults From 2001 to 2018. *The American Journal of Clinical Nutrition*, 115(1), 211–21. https://doi.org/10.1093/ajcn/nqab305

63. Wang, L., Martínez Steele, E., Du, M., Pomeranz, J. L., O'Connor, L. E., Herrick, K. A., Luo, H., Zhang, X., Mozaffarian, D., & Zhang, F. F. (2021). Trends in Consumption of Ultraprocessed Foods Among US Youths Aged 2–19 Years, 1999–2018. *JAMA*, 326(6), 519–30. https://doi.org/10.1001/jama.2021.10238

64. Franck, C., Grandi, S. M., & Eisenberg, M. J. (2013). Agricultural Subsidies and the American Obesity Epidemic. *American Journal of Preventive Medicine*, 45(3), 327–33. https://doi.org/10.1016/j.amepre.2013.04.010

65. Temple N. J. (2022). The Origins of the Obesity Epidemic in the USA—Lessons for Today. *Nutrients*, 14(20), 4253. https://doi.org/10.3390/nu14204253

66. Swinburn, B., Sacks, G., & Ravussin, E. (2009). Increased Food Energy Supply Is More Than Sufficient to Explain the US Epidemic of Obesity. *The American Journal of Clinical Nutrition*, 90(6), 1453–6. https://doi.org/10.3945/ajcn.2009.28595

67. Vandevijvere, S., Chow, C. C., Hall, K. D., Umali, E., & Swinburn, B. A. (2015). Increased Food Energy Supply as a Major Driver of the Obesity Epidemic: A Global Analysis. *Bulletin of the World Health Organization*, 93(7), 446–56. https://doi.org/10.2471/BLT.14.150565

68. Rao, M., Afshin, A., Singh, G., & Mozaffarian, D. (2013). Do Healthier Foods and Diet Patterns Cost More Than Less Healthy Options? A Systematic Review and Meta-Analysis. *BMJ Open*, 3(12), e004277. https://doi.org/10.1136/bmjopen-2013-004277

69. Darmon, N., & Drewnowski, A. (2015). Contribution of Food Prices and Diet Cost to Socioeconomic

Disparities in Diet Quality and Health: A Systematic Review and Analysis. *Nutrition Reviews*, 73(10), 643–60. https://doi.org/10.1093/nutrit/nuv027

70. Langfield, T., Marty, L., Inns, M., Jones, A., & Robinson, E. (2023). Healthier Diets for All? A Systematic Review and Meta-Analysis Examining Socioeconomic Equity of the Effect of Increasing Availability of Healthier Foods on Food Choice and Energy Intake. *Obesity Reviews: An Official Journal of the International Association for the Study of Obesity*, 24(6), e13565. https://doi.org/10.1111/obr.13565

71. Małachowska, A., & Jeżewska-Zychowicz, M. (2021). Does Examining the Childhood Food Experiences Help to Better Understand Food Choices in Adulthood? *Nutrients*, 13(3), 983. https://doi.org/10.3390/nu13030983

72. Telama, R., Yang, X., Viikari, J., Välimäki, I., Wanne, O., & Raitakari, O. (2005). Physical Activity From Childhood to Adulthood: A 21-Year Tracking Study. *American Journal of Preventive Medicine*, 28(3), 267–73. https://doi.org/10.1016/j.amepre.2004.12.003

73. Thedinga, H. K., Zehl, R., & Thiel, A. (2021). Weight Stigma Experiences and Self-Exclusion From Sport and Exercise Settings Among People With Obesity. *BMC Public Health*, 21(1), 565. https://doi.org/10.1186/s12889-021-10565-7

## Chapter 2

1. Anderson, J. W., Konz, E. C., Frederich, R. C., & Wood, C. L. (2001). Long-Term Weight Loss Maintenance: A Meta-Analysis of US Studies. *The American Journal of Clinical Nutrition*, 74(5), 579–84. https://doi.org/10.1093/ajcn/74.5.579

2. Nordmo, M., Danielsen, Y. S., & Nordmo, M. (2020). The Challenge of Keeping It Off, a Descriptive Systematic Review of High-Quality, Follow-Up Studies of Obesity Treatments. *Obesity Reviews: An Official Journal of the International Association for the Study of Obesity*, 21(1), e12949. https://doi.org/10.1111/obr.12949

3. Davenport, C. B. (1994). Body-Build and Its Inheritance. 1923. *Obesity Research*, 2(6), 606–23. https://doi.org/10.1002/j.1550-8528.1994.tb00112.x

4. Clark, P. J. (1956). The Heritability of Certain Anthropometric Characters As Ascertained From Measurements of Twins. *American Journal of Human Genetics*, 8(1), 49–54.

5. Osborne, R. H., & De George, F. V. (1959). *Genetic Basis of Morphological Variation: An*

*Evaluation and Application of the Twin Study Method.* Harvard University Press. https://doi.org/10.4159/harvard.9780674423312

6. Stunkard, A. J., Foch, T. T., & Hrubec, Z. (1986). A Twin Study of Human Obesity. *JAMA*, 256(1), 51–4. https://doi.org/10.1001/jama.1986.03380010055024

7. Stunkard, A. J., Harris, J. R., Pedersen, N. L., & McClearn, G. E. (1990). The Body-Mass Index of Twins Who Have Been Reared Apart. *The New England Journal of Medicine*, 322(21), 1483–87. https://doi.org/10.1056/NEJM199005243222102

8. Stunkard, A. J., Sørensen, T. I., Hanis, C., Teasdale, T. W., Chakraborty, R., Schull, W. J., & Schulsinger, F. (1986). An Adoption Study of Human Obesity. *The New England Journal of Medicine*, 314(4), 193–8. https://doi.org/10.1056/NEJM198601233140401

9. Price, R. A., Cadoret, R. J., Stunkard, A. J., & Troughton, E. (1987). Genetic Contributions to Human Fatness: An Adoption Study. *The American Journal of Psychiatry*, 144(8), 1003–8. https://doi.org/10.1176/ajp.144.8.1003

10. Ranadive, S. A., & Vaisse, C. (2008). Lessons From Extreme Human Obesity: Monogenic Disorders. *Endocrinology and Metabolism Clinics of North America*, 37(3), 733–X. https://doi.org/10.1016/j.ecl.2008.07.003

11. Mahmoud, R., Kimonis, V., & Butler, M. G. (2022). Genetics of Obesity in Humans: A Clinical Review. *International Journal of Molecular Sciences*, 23(19), 11005. https://doi.org/10.3390/ijms231911005

12. Hayashi, D., Edwards, C., Emond, J. A., Gilbert-Diamond, D., Butt, M., Rigby, A., & Masterson, T. D. (2023). What Is Food Noise? A Conceptual Model of Food Cue Reactivity. *Nutrients*, 15(22), 4809. https://doi.org/10.3390/nu15224809

13. Ramos, R. G., & Olden, K. (2008). Gene-Environment Interactions in the Development of Complex Disease Phenotypes. *International Journal of Environmental Research and Public Health*, 5(1), 4–11. https://doi.org/10.3390/ijerph5010004

14. Kennedy G. C. (1953). The Role of Depot Fat in the Hypothalamic Control of Food Intake in the Rat. *Proceedings of the Royal Society of London. Series B, Biological Sciences*, 140(901), 578–96. https://doi.org/10.1098/rspb.1953.0009

15. Guyenet, S. J., & Schwartz, M. W. (2012). Clinical Review: Regulation of Food Intake, Energy Balance, and Body Fat Mass: Implications for the Pathogenesis and Treatment of Obesity. *The Journal of Clinical Endocrinology and Metabolism*, 97(3), 745–55. https://doi.org/10.1210/jc.2011-2525

16. Speakman, J. R. (2018). The Evolution of Body Fatness:

Trading Off Disease and Predation Risk. *The Journal of Experimental Biology*, 221(Pt Suppl 1), jeb167254. https://doi.org/10.1242/jeb.167254

17. Thomas, J. G., Bond, D. S., Phelan, S., Hill, J. O., & Wing, R. R. (2014). Weight Loss Maintenance for 10 Years in the National Weight Control Registry. *American Journal of Preventive Medicine*, 46(1), 17–23. https://doi.org/10.1016/j.amepre.2013.08.019

18. Speakman, J. R., & Hall, K. D. (2023). Models of Body Weight and Fatness Regulation. *Philosophical Transactions of the Royal Society of London. Series B, Biological Sciences*, 378(1888), 20220231. https://doi.org/10.1098/rstb.2022.0231

19. Lund, J., & Clemmensen, C. (2023). Physiological Protection Against Weight Gain: Evidence From Overfeeding Studies and Future Directions. *Philosophical Transactions of the Royal Society of London. Series B, Biological Sciences*, 378(1885), 20220229. https://doi.org/10.1098/rstb.2022.0229

20. Polidori, D., Sanghvi, A., Seeley, R. J., & Hall, K. D. (2016). How Strongly Does Appetite Counter Weight Loss? Quantification of the Feedback Control of Human Energy Intake. Obesity (Silver Spring, Md.), 24(11), 2289–2295. https://doi.org/10.1002/oby.21653

21. Sumithran, P., Prendergast, L. A., Delbridge, E., Purcell, K., Shulkes, A., Kriketos, A., & Proietto, J. (2011). Long-Term Persistence of Hormonal Adaptations to Weight Loss. *The New England Journal of Medicine*, 365(17), 1597–1604. https://doi.org/10.1056/NEJMoa1105816

22. Müller, M. J., Enderle, J., & Bosy-Westphal, A. (2016). Changes in Energy Expenditure With Weight Gain and Weight Loss in Humans. *Current Obesity Reports*, 5(4), 413–23. https://doi.org/10.1007/s13679-016-0237-4

23. Ravussin, E., Smith, S. R., & Ferrante, A. W., Jr.. (2021). Physiology of Energy Expenditure in the Weight-Reduced State. *Obesity*, 29 Suppl 1, S31–8. https://doi.org/10.1002/oby.23095

24. Hall, K. D. (2024). Physiology of the Weight loss Plateau in Response to Diet Restriction, GLP1 Receptor Agonism, and Bariatric Surgery. *Obesity*, 32(6), 1163–68. https://doi.org/10.1002/oby.24027

25. Wilding, J. P. H., Batterham, R. L., Davies, M., Van Gaal, L. F., Kandler, K., Konakli, K., Lingvay, I., McGowan, B. M., Oral, T. K., Rosenstock, J., Wadden, T. A., Wharton, S., Yokote, K., Kushner, R. F., & STEP 1 Study Group (2022). Weight Regain and Cardiometabolic Effects After Withdrawal of Semaglutide: The Step 1 Trial Extension. *Diabetes, Obesity & Metabolism*, 24(8), 1553–64. https://doi.org/10.1111/dom.14725

26. Noria, S. F., Shelby, R. D., Atkins, K. D., Nguyen, N. T., & Gadde, K. M. (2023). Weight Regain After Bariatric Surgery: Scope of the Problem, Causes, Prevention, and Treatment. *Current Diabetes Reports*, 23(3), 31–42. https://doi.org/10.1007/s11892-023-01498-z

27. Wilding, J. P. H. et al. Weight Regain and Cardiometabolic Effects After Withdrawal of Semaglutide.

28. Eskandari, F., Lake, A. A., Rose, K., Butler, M., & O'Malley, C. (2022). A Mixed-Method Systematic Review and Meta-Analysis of the Influences of Food Environments and Food Insecurity on Obesity in High-Income Countries. *Food Science & Nutrition*, 10(11), 3689–723. https://doi.org/10.1002/fsn3.2969

29. Atanasova, P., Kusuma, D., Pineda, E., Frost, G., Sassi, F., & Miraldo, M. (2022). The Impact of the Consumer and Neighbourhood Food Environment on Dietary Intake and Obesity-Related Outcomes: A Systematic Review of Causal Impact Studies. *Social Science & Medicine*, 299, 114879. https://doi.org/10.1016/j.socscimed.2022.114879

30. Dakanalis, A., Mentzelou, M., Papadopoulou, S. K., Papandreou, D., Spanoudaki, M., Vasios, G. K., Pavlidou, E., Mantzorou, M., & Giaginis, C. (2023). The Association of Emotional Eating With Overweight/Obesity, Depression, Anxiety/Stress, and Dietary Patterns: A Review of the Current Clinical Evidence. *Nutrients*, 15(5), 1173. https://doi.org/10.3390/nu15051173

31. Mannan, M., Mamun, A., Doi, S., & Clavarino, A. (2016). Is There a Bi-directional Relationship Between Depression and Obesity Among Adult Men and Women? Systematic Review and Bias-Adjusted Meta Analysis. *Asian Journal of Psychiatry*, 21, 51–66. https://doi.org/10.1016/j.ajp.2015.12.008

32. Afzal, M., Siddiqi, N., Ahmad, B., Afsheen, N., Aslam, F., Ali, A., Ayesha, R., Bryant, M., Holt, R., Khalid, H., Ishaq, K., Koly, K. N., Rajan, S., Saba, J., Tirbhowan, N., & Zavala, G. A. (2021). Prevalence of Overweight and Obesity in People With Severe Mental Illness: Systematic Review and Meta-Analysis. *Frontiers in Endocrinology*, 12, 769309. https://doi.org/10.3389/fendo.2021.769309

33. World Health Organization (2023). WHO Acceleration Plan to Stop Obesity. Retrieved from https://iris.who.int/bitstream/handle/10665/370281/9789240075634-eng.pdf

34. Foster, G. D., Wadden, T. A., Vogt, R. A., & Brewer, G. (1997). What Is a Reasonable Weight Loss? Patients' Expectations and Evaluations of Obesity Treatment Outcomes. *Journal of Consulting and Clinical*

*Psychology*, 65(1), 79–85. https://doi.org/10.1037/0022-006x.65.1.79

35. Pétré, B., Scheen, A., Ziegler, O., Donneau, A. F., Dardenne, N., Husson, E., Albert, A., & Guillaume, M. (2018). Weight Loss Expectations and Determinants in a Large Community-Based Sample. *Preventive Medicine Reports*, 12, 12–19. https://doi.org/10.1016/j.pmedr.2018.08.005

36. Ferraro, Z. M., Patterson, S., & Chaput, J. P. (2015). Unhealthy Weight Control Practices: Culprits and Clinical Recommendations. *Clinical Medicine Insights: Endocrinology and Diabetes*, 8, 7–11. https://doi.org/10.4137/CMED.S23060

37. Neumark-Sztainer, D., Wall, M., Story, M., & Standish, A. R. (2012). Dieting and Unhealthy Weight Control Behaviors During Adolescence: Associations With 10-Year Changes in Body Mass Index. *The Journal of Adolescent Health: Official Publication of the Society for Adolescent Medicine*, 50(1), 80–6. https://doi.org/10.1016/j.jadohealth.2011.05.010

38. Neumark-Sztainer, D. R., Wall, M. M., Haines, J. I., Story, M. T., Sherwood, N. E., & Van Den Berg, P. A. (2007). Shared Risk and Protective Factors for Overweight and Disordered Eating in Adolescents. *American Journal of Preventive Medicine*, 33(5), 359–69. https://doi.org/10.1016/j.amepre.2007.07.031

39. Chaitoff, A., Swetlik, C., Ituarte, C., Pfoh, E., Lee, L. L., Heinberg, L. J., & Rothberg, M. B. (2019). Associations Between Unhealthy Weight Loss Strategies and Depressive Symptoms. *American Journal of Preventive Medicine*, 56(2), 241–50. https://doi.org/10.1016/j.amepre.2018.09.017

40. Crow, S., Eisenberg, M. E., Story, M., & Neumark-Sztainer, D. (2008). Suicidal Behavior in Adolescents: Relationship to Weight Status, Weight Control Behaviors, and Body Dissatisfaction. *The International Journal of Eating Disorders*, 41(1), 82–7. https://doi.org/10.1002/eat.20466

41. Golay, A., Buclin, S., Ybarra, J., Toti, F., Pichard, C., Picco, N., de Tonnac, N., & Allaz, A. F. (2004). New Interdisciplinary Cognitive-Behavioural-Nutritional Approach to Obesity Treatment: A 5-Year Follow-Up Study. *Eating and Weight Disorders—Studies on Anorexia, Bulimia, and Obesity*, 9(1), 29–34. https://doi.org/10.1007/BF03325042

42. Look Ahead Research Group (2014). Eight-Year Weight Losses With an Intensive Lifestyle Intervention: The Look Ahead Study. *Obesity*, 22(1), 5–13. https://doi.org/10.1002/oby.20662

43. Stunkard, A., & McLaren-Hume, M. (1959). The Results of Treatment for Obesity: A Review of the Literature and Report of a Series. *A.M.A. Archives of Internal Medicine*, 103(1), 79–85. https://doi.org/10.1001/archinte.1959.00270010085011

44. Golay, A. et al. New Interdisciplinary Cognitive-Behavioural-Nutritional Approach to Obesity Treatment.

45. Look Ahead Research Group. Eight-Year Weight Losses With an Intensive Lifestyle Intervention.

46. Binsaeed, B., Aljohani, F. G., Alsobiai, F. F., Alraddadi, M., Alrehaili, A. A., Alnahdi, B. S., Almotairi, F. S., Jumah, M. A., & Alrehaili, A. T. (2023). Barriers and Motivators to Weight Loss in People With Obesity. *Cureus*, 15(11), e49040. https://doi.org/10.7759/cureus.49040

47. Tay, A., Hoeksema, H., & Murphy, R. (2023). Uncovering Barriers and Facilitators of Weight Loss and Weight Loss Maintenance: Insights From Qualitative Research. *Nutrients*, 15(5), 1297. https://doi.org/10.3390/nu15051297

48. Deslippe, A. L., Soanes, A., Bouchaud, C. C., Beckenstein, H., Slim, M., Plourde, H., & Cohen, T. R. (2023). Barriers and Facilitators to Diet, Physical Activity and Lifestyle Behavior Intervention Adherence: A Qualitative Systematic Review of the Literature. *The International Journal of Behavioral Nutrition and Physical Activity*, 20(1), 14. https://doi.org/10.1186/s12966-023-01424-2

49. Silva, D. F. O., Sena-Evangelista, K. C. M., Lyra, C. O., Pedrosa, L. F. C., Arrais, R. F., & Lima, S. C. V. C. (2018). Motivations for Weight Loss in Adolescents With Overweight and Obesity: A Systematic Review. *BMC Pediatrics*, 18(1), 364. https://doi.org/10.1186/s12887-018-1333-2

50. Kelly, S., Martin, S., Kuhn, I., Cowan, A., Brayne, C., & Lafortune, L. (2016). Barriers and Facilitators to the Uptake and Maintenance of Healthy Behaviours by People at Mid-Life: A Rapid Systematic Review. *PloS One*, 11(1), e0145074. https://doi.org/10.1371/journal.pone.0145074

51. Guess, N. (2012). A Qualitative Investigation of Attitudes Towards Aerobic and Resistance Exercise Amongst Overweight and Obese Individuals. *BMC Research Notes*, 5, 191. https://doi.org/10.1186/1756-0500-5-191

52. de Jong, M., Jansen, N., & van Middelkoop, M. (2023). A Systematic Review of Patient Barriers and Facilitators for Implementing Lifestyle Interventions Targeting Weight Loss in Primary Care. *Obesity Reviews: An Official Journal of the International Association for the Study of Obesity*, 24(8), e13571. https://doi.org/10.1111/obr.13571

53. McCormack, G. R., McFadden, K., McHugh, T. L. F., Spence, J. C., & Mummery, K. (2019). Barriers and Facilitators Impacting the Experiences of Adults Participating in an Internet-Facilitated Pedometer Intervention. *Psychology of Sport and Exercise*, 45, 101549. https://doi.org/10.1016/j.psychsport.2019.101549

54. Korkiakangas, E. E., Alahuhta, M. A., Husman, P. M., Keinänen-Kiukaanniemi, S., Taanila, A. M., & Laitinen, J. H. (2011). Motivators and Barriers to Exercise Among Adults With a High Risk of Type 2 Diabetes—a Qualitative Study. *Scandinavian Journal of Caring Sciences*, 25(1), 62–9. https://doi.org/10.1111/j.1471-6712.2010.00791.x

55. Wycherley, T. P., Mohr, P., Noakes, M., Clifton, P. M., & Brinkworth, G. D. (2012). Self-Reported Facilitators of, and Impediments to Maintenance of Healthy Lifestyle Behaviours Following a Supervised Research-Based Lifestyle Intervention Programme in Patients With Type 2 Diabetes. *Diabetic Medicine: A Journal of the British Diabetic Association*, 29(5), 632–9. https://doi.org/10.1111/j.1464-5491.2011.03451.x

56. Burke, L. E., Swigart, V., Warziski Turk, M., Derro, N., & Ewing, L. J. (2009). Experiences of Self-Monitoring: Successes and Struggles During Treatment for Weight Loss. *Qualitative Health Research*, 19(6), 815–28. https://doi.org/10.1177/1049732309335395

57. Cooke, A. B., Pace, R., Chan, D., Rosenberg, E., Dasgupta, K., & Daskalopoulou, S. S. (2018). A Qualitative Evaluation of a Physician-Delivered Pedometer-Based Step Count Prescription Strategy With Insight From Participants and Treating Physicians. *Diabetes Research and Clinical Practice*, 139, 314–22. https://doi.org/10.1016/j.diabres.2018.03.008

## Chapter 3

1. Johnston, B. C., Kanters, S., Bandayrel, K., Wu, P., Naji, F., Siemieniuk, R. A., Ball, G. D., Busse, J. W., Thorlund, K., Guyatt, G., Jansen, J. P., & Mills, E. J. (2014). Comparison of Weight Loss Among Named Diet Programs in Overweight and Obese Adults: A Meta-Analysis. *JAMA*, 312(9), 923–33. https://doi.org/10.1001/jama.2014.10397

2. Ibid.

3. Ge, L., Sadeghirad, B., Ball, G. D. C., da Costa, B. R., Hitchcock, C. L., Svendrovski, A., Kiflen, R., Quadri, K., Kwon, H. Y., Karamouzian, M., Adams-Webber, T., Ahmed, W., Damanhoury, S., Zeraatkar, D., Nikolakopoulou, A., Tsuyuki, R. T., Tian, J., Yang, K., Guyatt, G. H., & Johnston, B. C. (2020). Comparison of Dietary Macronutrient Patterns

of 14 Popular Named Dietary Programmes for Weight and Cardiovascular Risk Factor Reduction in Adults: Systematic Review and Network Meta-Analysis of Randomised Trials. *BMJ*, 369, m696. https://doi.org/10.1136/bmj.m696

4. Elortegui Pascual, P., Rolands, M. R., Eldridge, A. L., Kassis, A., Mainardi, F., Lê, K. A., Karagounis, L. G., Gut, P., & Varady, K. A. (2023). A Meta-Analysis Comparing the Effectiveness of Alternate Day Fasting, the 5:2 Diet, and Time-Restricted Eating for Weight Loss. *Obesity*, 31 Suppl 1(Suppl 1), 9–21. https://doi.org/10.1002/oby.23568

5. Churuangsuk, C., Hall, J., Reynolds, A., Griffin, S. J., Combet, E., & Lean, M. E. J. (2022). Diets for Weight Management in Adults With Type 2 Diabetes: An Umbrella Review of Published Meta-Analyses and Systematic Review of Trials of Diets for Diabetes Remission. *Diabetologia*, 65(1), 14–36. https://doi.org/10.1007/s00125-021-05577-2

6. Dansinger, M. L., Gleason, J. A., Griffith, J. L., Selker, H. P., & Schaefer, E. J. (2005). Comparison of the Atkins, Ornish, Weight Watchers, and Zone Diets for Weight Loss and Heart Disease Risk Reduction: A Randomized Trial. *JAMA*, 293(1), 43–53. https://doi.org/10.1001/jama.293.1.43

7. Anton, S. D., Hida, A., Heekin, K., Sowalsky, K., Karabetian, C., Mutchie, H., Leeuwenburgh, C., Manini, T. M., & Barnett, T. E. (2017). Effects of Popular Diets Without Specific Calorie Targets on Weight Loss Outcomes: Systematic Review of Findings From Clinical Trials. *Nutrients*, 9(8), 822. https://doi.org/10.3390/nu9080822

8. Ludwig, D. S., & Ebbeling, C. B. (2018). The Carbohydrate-Insulin Model of Obesity: Beyond "Calories In, Calories Out." *JAMA Internal Medicine*, 178(8), 1098–103. https://doi.org/10.1001/jamainternmed.2018.2933

9. Ludwig, D. S., Aronne, L. J., Astrup, A., de Cabo, R., Cantley, L. C., Friedman, M. I., Heymsfield, S. B., Johnson, J. D., King, J. C., Krauss, R. M., Lieberman, D. E., Taubes, G., Volek, J. S., Westman, E. C., Willett, W. C., Yancy, W. S., & Ebbeling, C. B. (2021). The Carbohydrate-Insulin Model: A Physiological Perspective on the Obesity Pandemic. *The American Journal of Clinical Nutrition*, 114(6), 1873–85. https://doi.org/10.1093/ajcn/nqab270

10. Ludwig, D. S., Apovian, C. M., Aronne, L. J., Astrup, A., Cantley, L. C., Ebbeling, C. B., Heymsfield, S. B., Johnson, J. D., King, J. C., Krauss, R. M., Taubes, G., Volek, J. S., Westman, E. C., Willett, W. C., Yancy, W. S., Jr., & Friedman, M. I. (2022). Competing Paradigms

of Obesity Pathogenesis: Energy Balance Versus Carbohydrate-Insulin Models. *European Journal of Clinical Nutrition*, 76(9), 1209–21. https://doi.org/10.1038/s41430-022-01179-2

11. Anton, S. D. et al. Effects of Popular Diets Without Specific Calorie Targets on Weight Loss Outcomes.

12. Willems, A. E. M., Sura-De Jong, M., Van Beek, A. P., Nederhof, E., & Van Dijk, G. (2021). Effects of Macronutrient Intake in Obesity: A Meta-Analysis of Low-Carbohydrate and Low-Fat Diets on Markers of the Metabolic Syndrome. *Nutrition Reviews*, 79(4), 429–44. https://doi.org/10.1093/nutrit/nuaa044

13. Hansen, T. T., Astrup, A., & Sjödin, A. (2021). Are Dietary Proteins the Key to Successful Body Weight Management? A Systematic Review and Meta-Analysis of Studies Assessing Body Weight Outcomes After Interventions With Increased Dietary Protein. *Nutrients*, 13(9), 3193. https://doi.org/10.3390/nu13093193

14. Tagawa, R., Watanabe, D., Ito, K., Ueda, K., Nakayama, K., Sanbongi, C., & Miyachi, M. (2020). Dose-Response Relationship Between Protein Intake and Muscle Mass Increase: A Systematic Review and Meta-Analysis of Randomized Controlled Trials. *Nutrition Reviews*, 79(1), 66–75. https://doi.org/10.1093/nutrit/nuaa104

15. Yang, M. U., & Van Itallie, T. B. (1976). Composition of Weight Lost During Short-Term Weight Reduction. Metabolic Responses of Obese Subjects to Starvation and Low-Calorie Ketogenic and Nonketogenic Diets. *The Journal of Clinical Investigation*, 58(3), 722–30. https://doi.org/10.1172/JCI108519

16. Hall, K. D., & Guo, J. (2017). Obesity Energetics: Body Weight Regulation and the Effects of Diet Composition. *Gastroenterology*, 152(7), 1718–27.e3. https://doi.org/10.1053/j.gastro.2017.01.052

17. Churuangsuk, C., Kherouf, M., Combet, E., & Lean, M. (2018). Low-Carbohydrate Diets for Overweight and Obesity: A Systematic Review of the Systematic Reviews. *Obesity Reviews: An Official Journal of the International Association for the Study of Obesity*, 19(12), 1700–18. https://doi.org/10.1111/obr.12744

18. Ge, L. et al. Comparison of Dietary Macronutrient Patterns of 14 Popular Named Dietary Programmes for Weight and Cardiovascular Risk Factor Reduction in Adults.

19. Tobias, D. K., Chen, M., Manson, J. E., Ludwig, D. S., Willett, W., & Hu, F. B. (2015). Effect of Low-Fat Diet Interventions Versus Other Diet Interventions on Long-Term Weight Change in Adults: A Systematic Review and Meta-Analysis. *The Lancet: Diabetes*

& *Endocrinology*, 3(12), 968–79. https://doi.org/10.1016/S2213-8587(15)00367-8

20. Rolls, B. J. (2017). Dietary Energy Density: Applying Behavioural Science to Weight Management. *Nutrition Bulletin*, 42(3), 246–53. https://doi.org/10.1111/nbu.12280

21. Lissner, L., Levitsky, D. A., Strupp, B. J., Kalkwarf, H. J., & Roe, D. A. (1987). Dietary Fat and the Regulation of Energy Intake in Human Subjects. *The American Journal of Clinical Nutrition*, 46(6), 886–92. https://doi.org/10.1093/ajcn/46.6.886

22. Kendall, A., Levitsky, D. A., Strupp, B. J., & Lissner, L. (1991). Weight Loss on a Low-Fat Diet: Consequence of the Imprecision of the Control of Food Intake in Humans. *The American Journal of Clinical Nutrition*, 53(5), 1124–9. https://doi.org/10.1093/ajcn/53.5.1124

23. Hall, K. D., & Guo, J. Obesity Energetics.

24. Ibid.

25. Ge, L. et al. Comparison of Dietary Macronutrient Patterns of 14 Popular Named Dietary Programmes for Weight and Cardiovascular Risk Factor Reduction in Adults.

26. Wycherley, T. P., Moran, L. J., Clifton, P. M., Noakes, M., & Brinkworth, G. D. (2012). Effects of Energy-Restricted High-Protein, Low-Fat Compared With Standard-Protein, Low-Fat Diets: A Meta-Analysis of Randomized Controlled Trials. *The American Journal of Clinical Nutrition*, 96(6), 1281–98. https://doi.org/10.3945/ajcn.112.044321

27. Leidy, H. J., Clifton, P. M., Astrup, A., Wycherley, T. P., Westerterp-Plantenga, M. S., Luscombe-Marsh, N. D., Woods, S. C., & Mattes, R. D. (2015). The Role of Protein in Weight Loss and Maintenance. *The American Journal of Clinical Nutrition*, 101(6), 1320–9S. https://doi.org/10.3945/ajcn.114.084038

28. Hudson, J. L., Wang, Y., Bergia, R. E., III, & Campbell, W. W. (2020). Protein Intake Greater Than the RDA Differentially Influences Whole-Body Lean Mass Responses to Purposeful Catabolic and Anabolic Stressors: A Systematic Review and Meta-Analysis. *Advances in Nutrition*, 11(3), 548–58. https://doi.org/10.1093/advances/nmz106

29. Strasser, B., Volaklis, K., Fuchs, D., & Burtscher, M. (2018). Role of Dietary Protein and Muscular Fitness on Longevity and Aging. *Aging and Disease*, 9(1), 119–32. https://doi.org/10.14336/AD.2017.0202

30. Moon, J., & Koh, G. (2020). Clinical Evidence and Mechanisms of High-Protein Diet-Induced Weight Loss. *Journal of Obesity & Metabolic Syndrome*, 29(3), 166–73. https://doi.org/10.7570/jomes20028

31. Kohanmoo, A., Faghih, S., & Akhlaghi, M. (2020). Effect of Short- and Long-Term Protein Consumption on Appetite and Appetite-Regulating Gastrointestinal Hormones, a Systematic Review and Meta-Analysis of Randomized Controlled Trials. *Physiology & Behavior*, 226, 113123. https://doi.org/10.1016/j.physbeh.2020.113123

32. Hall, K. D., & Guo, J., Obesity Energetics.

33. Ventriglio, A., Sancassiani, F., Contu, M. P., Latorre, M., Di Slavatore, M., Fornaro, M., & Bhugra, D. (2020). Mediterranean Diet and Its Benefits on Health and Mental Health: A Literature Review. *Clinical Practice and Epidemiology in Mental Health*, 16(Suppl-1), 156–64. https://doi.org/10.2174/1745017902016010156

34. Papadaki, A., Nolen-Doerr, E., & Mantzoros, C. S. (2020). The Effect of the Mediterranean Diet on Metabolic Health: A Systematic Review and Meta-Analysis of Controlled Trials in Adults. *Nutrients*, 12(11), 3342. https://doi.org/10.3390/nu12113342

35. Dinu, M., Pagliai, G., Casini, A., & Sofi, F. (2018). Mediterranean Diet and Multiple Health Outcomes: An Umbrella Review of Meta-Analyses of Observational Studies and Randomised Trials. *European Journal of Clinical Nutrition*, 72(1), 30–43. https://doi.org/10.1038/ejcn.2017.58

36. Soltani, S., Jayedi, A., Shab-Bidar, S., Becerra-Tomás, N., & Salas-Salvadó, J. (2019). Adherence to the Mediterranean Diet in Relation to All-Cause Mortality: A Systematic Review and Dose-Response Meta-Analysis of Prospective Cohort Studies. *Advances in Nutrition*, 10(6), 1029–39. https://doi.org/10.1093/advances/nmz041

37. Schwingshackl, L., Morze, J., & Hoffmann, G. (2020). Mediterranean Diet and Health Status: Active Ingredients and Pharmacological Mechanisms. *British Journal of Pharmacology*, 177(6), 1241–57. https://doi.org/10.1111/bph.14778

38. Hall, K. D., et al. Ultra-Processed Diets Cause Excess Calorie Intake and Weight Gain.

39. Mancini, J. G., Filion, K. B., Atallah, R., & Eisenberg, M. J. (2016). Systematic Review of the Mediterranean Diet for Long-Term Weight Loss. *The American Journal of Medicine*, 129(4), 407–15.e4. https://doi.org/10.1016/j.amjmed.2015.11.028

40. Appel, L. J., Moore, T. J., Obarzanek, E., Vollmer, W. M., Svetkey, L. P., Sacks, F. M., Bray, G. A., Vogt, T. M., Cutler, J. A., Windhauser, M. M., Lin, P. H., & Karanja, N. (1997). A Clinical Trial of the Effects of Dietary Patterns on Blood Pressure. DASH Collaborative Research Group. *The New England Journal of Medicine*, 336(16),

1117–24. https://doi.org/10.1056/
NEJM199704173361601

41. NCD Risk Factor Collaboration
(NCD-RisC) (2021). Worldwide
Trends in Hypertension
Prevalence and Progress in
Treatment and Control From 1990
to 2019: A Pooled Analysis of 1201
Population-Representative Studies
With 104 Million Participants. *The
Lancet*, 398(10304), 957–80. https://
doi.org/10.1016/S0140-6736(21)
01330-1

42. Carey, R. M., Moran, A. E., &
Whelton, P. K. (2022). Treatment
of Hypertension: A Review. *JAMA*,
328(18), 1849–61. https://doi.
org/10.1001/jama.2022.19590

43. Appel, L. J. et al. A Clinical Trial
of the Effects of Dietary Patterns
on Blood Pressure.

44. Ibid.

45. Sacks, F. M., Svetkey, L. P.,
Vollmer, W. M., Appel, L. J., Bray,
G. A., Harsha, D., Obarzanek,
E., Conlin, P. R., Miller, E. R., III,
Simons-Morton, D. G., Karanja,
N., Lin, P. H., & DASH-Sodium
Collaborative Research Group
(2001). Effects on Blood Pressure
of Reduced Dietary Sodium and
the Dietary Approaches to Stop
Hypertension (DASH) Diet.
DASH-Sodium Collaborative
Research Group. *The New England
Journal of Medicine*, 344(1),
3–10. https://doi.org/10.1056/
NEJM200101043440101

46. Appel, L. J., Sacks, F. M., Carey,
V. J., Obarzanek, E., Swain, J. F.,

Miller, E. R., III, Conlin, P. R.,
Erlinger, T. P., Rosner, B. A.,
Laranjo, N. M., Charleston, J.,
McCarron, P., Bishop, L. M.,
& OmniHeart Collaborative
Research Group (2005). Effects
of Protein, Monounsaturated
Fat, and Carbohydrate Intake
on Blood Pressure and Serum
Lipids: Results of the OmniHeart
Randomized Trial. *JAMA*, 294(19),
2455–64. https://doi.org/10.1001/
jama.294.19.2455

47. Sacks, F. M., Carey, V. J., Anderson,
C. A., Miller, E. R., III, Copeland,
T., Charleston, J., Harshfield, B. J.,
Laranjo, N., McCarron, P., Swain,
J., White, K., Yee, K., & Appel,
L. J. (2014). Effects of High vs
Low Glycemic Index of Dietary
Carbohydrate on Cardiovascular
Disease Risk Factors and Insulin
Sensitivity: The OmniCarb
Randomized Clinical Trial.
*JAMA*, 312(23), 2531–41. https://doi.
org/10.1001/jama.2014.16658

48. Lari, A., Sohouli, M. H., Fatahi,
S., Cerqueira, H. S., Santos, H. O.,
Pourrajab, B., Rezaei, M., Saneie,
S., & Rahideh, S. T. (2021). The
Effects of the Dietary Approaches
to Stop Hypertension (DASH)
Diet on Metabolic Risk Factors in
Patients With Chronic Disease:
A Systematic Review and
Meta-Analysis of Randomized
Controlled Trials. *Nutrition,
Metabolism, and Cardiovascular
Diseases: NMCD*, 31(10),

2766–78. https://doi.org/10.1016/j. numecd.2021.05.030

49. Cordain, L., Eaton, S. B., Sebastian, A., Mann, N., Lindeberg, S., Watkins, B. A., O'Keefe, J. H., & Brand-Miller, J. (2005). Origins and Evolution of the Western Diet: Health Implications for the 21st Century. *The American Journal of Clinical Nutrition*, 81(2), 341–54. https://doi.org/10.1093/ ajcn.81.2.341

50. Ibid.

51. Genoni, A., Lo, J., Lyons-Wall, P., & Devine, A. (2016). Compliance, Palatability and Feasibility of Paleolithic and Australian Guide to Healthy Eating Diets in Healthy Women: A 4-Week Dietary Intervention. *Nutrients*, 8(8), 481. https://doi.org/10.3390/ nu8080481

52. Hall, K. D., et al. Ultra-Processed Diets Cause Excess Calorie Intake and Weight Gain.

53. de Menezes, E. V. A., Sampaio, H. A. C., Carioca, A. A. F., Parente, N. A., Brito, F. O., Moreira, T. M. M., de Souza, A. C. C., & Arruda, S. P. M. (2019). Influence of Paleolithic Diet on Anthropometric Markers in Chronic Diseases: Systematic Review and Meta-Analysis. *Nutrition Journal*, 18(1), 41. https://doi.org/10.1186/ s12937-019-0457-z

54. Ghaedi, E., Mohammadi, M., Mohammadi, H., Ramezani-Jolfaie, N., Malekzadeh, J.,

Hosseinzadeh, M., & Salehi-Abargouei, A. (2019). Effects of a Paleolithic Diet on Cardiovascular Disease Risk Factors: A Systematic Review and Meta-Analysis of Randomized Controlled Trials. *Advances in Nutrition*, 10(4), 634–46. https://doi.org/10.1093/ advances/nmz007

55. Manheimer, E. W., van Zuuren, E. J., Fedorowicz, Z., & Pijl, H. (2015). Paleolithic Nutrition for Metabolic Syndrome: Systematic Review and Meta-Analysis. *The American Journal of Clinical Nutrition*, 102(4), 922–32. https:// doi.org/10.3945/ajcn.115.113613

56. Liang, S., Mijatovic, J., Li, A., Koemel, N., Nasir, R., Toniutti, C., Bell-Anderson, K., Skilton, M., & O'Leary, F. (2022). Dietary Patterns and Non-communicable Disease Biomarkers: A Network Meta-Analysis and Nutritional Geometry Approach. *Nutrients*, 15(1), 76. https://doi.org/10.3390/ nu15010076

57. Parker, H. W., & Vadiveloo, M. K. (2019). Diet Quality of Vegetarian Diets Compared With Nonvegetarian Diets: A Systematic Review. *Nutrition Reviews*, 77(3), 144–60. https://doi.org/10.1093/ nutrit/nuy067

58. Oussalah, A., Levy, J., Berthezène, C., Alpers, D. H., & Guéant, J. L. (2020). Health Outcomes Associated With Vegetarian Diets: An Umbrella Review of Systematic Reviews and Meta-Analyses.

*Clinical Nutrition*, 39(11), 3283–307. https://doi.org/10.1016/j.clnu.2020.02.037

59. Wang, T., Kroeger, C. M., Cassidy, S., Mitra, S., Ribeiro, R. V., Jose, S., Masedunskas, A., Senior, A. M., & Fontana, L. (2023). Vegetarian Dietary Patterns and Cardiometabolic Risk in People With or at High Risk of Cardiovascular Disease: A Systematic Review and Meta-Analysis. *JAMA Network Open*, 6(7), e2325658. https://doi.org/10.1001/jamanetworkopen.2023.25658

60. Landry, M. J., Ward, C. P., Cunanan, K. M., Durand, L. R., Perelman, D., Robinson, J. L., Hennings, T., Koh, L., Dant, C., Zeitlin, A., Ebel, E. R., Sonnenburg, E. D., Sonnenburg, J. L., & Gardner, C. D. (2023). Cardiometabolic Effects of Omnivorous vs Vegan Diets in Identical Twins: A Randomized Clinical Trial. *JAMA Network Open*, 6(11), e2344457. https://doi.org/10.1001/jamanetworkopen.2023.44457

61. Chew, H. S. J., Heng, F. K. X., Tien, S. A., Thian, J. Y., Chou, H. S., Loong, S. S. E., Ang, W. H. D., Chew, N. W. S., & Lo, K. K. (2023). Effects of Plant-Based Diets on Anthropometric and Cardiometabolic Markers in Adults: An Umbrella Review. *Nutrients*, 15(10), 2331. https://doi.org/10.3390/nu15102331

62. Selinger, E., Neuenschwander, M., Koller, A., Gojda, J., Kühn, T., Schwingshackl, L., Barbaresko, J., & Schlesinger, S. (2023). Evidence of a Vegan Diet for Health Benefits and Risks—an Umbrella Review of Meta-Analyses of Observational and Clinical Studies. *Critical Reviews in Food Science and Nutrition*, 63(29), 9926–36. https://doi.org/10.1080/10408398.2022.2075311

63. Pawlak, R., Lester, S. E., & Babatunde, T. (2014). The Prevalence of Cobalamin Deficiency Among Vegetarians Assessed by Serum Vitamin B12: A Review of Literature. *European Journal of Clinical Nutrition*, 68(5), 541–8. https://doi.org/10.1038/ejcn.2014.46

64. Bakaloudi, D. R., Halloran, A., Rippin, H. L., Oikonomidou, A. C., Dardavesis, T. I., Williams, J., Wickramasinghe, K., Breda, J., & Chourdakis, M. (2021). Intake and Adequacy of the Vegan Diet. A Systematic Review of the Evidence. *Clinical Nutrition*, 40(5), 3503–21. https://doi.org/10.1016/j.clnu.2020.11.035

65. Hevia-Larraín, V., Gualano, B., Longobardi, I., Gil, S., Fernandes, A. L., Costa, L. A. R., Pereira, R. M. R., Artioli, G. G., Phillips, S. M., & Roschel, H. (2021). High-Protein Plant-Based Diet Versus a Protein-Matched Omnivorous Diet to Support Resistance Training Adaptations:

A Comparison Between Habitual Vegans and Omnivores. *Sports Medicine*, 51(6), 1317–30. https://doi.org/10.1007/s40279-021-01434-9

66. Judge, A., & Dodd, M. S. (2020). Metabolism. *Essays in Biochemistry*, 64(4), 607–47. https://doi.org/10.1042/EBC20190041

67. Fernando, H. A., Zibellini, J., Harris, R. A., Seimon, R. V., & Sainsbury, A. (2019). Effect of Ramadan Fasting on Weight and Body Composition in Healthy Non-athlete Adults: A Systematic Review and Meta-Analysis. *Nutrients*, 11(2), 478. https://doi.org/10.3390/nu11020478

68. Jahrami, H., Trabelsi, K., Alhaj, O. A., Saif, Z., Pandi-Perumal, S. R., & BaHammam, A. S. (2022). The Impact of Ramadan Fasting on the Metabolic Syndrome Severity in Relation to Ethnicity and Sex: Results of a Systematic Review and Meta-Analysis. *Nutrition, Metabolism, and Cardiovascular Diseases: NMCD*, 32(12), 2714–29. https://doi.org/10.1016/j.numecd.2022.09.001

69. Huang, L., Chen, Y., Wen, S., Lu, D., Shen, X., Deng, H., & Xu, L. (2022). Is Time-Restricted Eating (8/16) Beneficial for Body Weight and Metabolism of Obese and Overweight Adults? A Systematic Review and Meta-Analysis of Randomized Controlled Trials. *Food Science & Nutrition*, 11(3), 1187–200. https://doi.org/10.1002/fsn3.3194

70. Sievert, K., Hussain, S. M., Page, M. J., Wang, Y., Hughes, H. J., Malek, M., & Cicuttini, F. M. (2019). Effect of Breakfast on Weight and Energy Intake: Systematic Review and Meta-Analysis of Randomised Controlled Trials. *BMJ*, 364, l42. https://doi.org/10.1136/bmj.l42

71. Ma, X., Chen, Q., Pu, Y., Guo, M., Jiang, Z., Huang, W., Long, Y., & Xu, Y. (2020). Skipping Breakfast Is Associated With Overweight and Obesity: A Systematic Review and Meta-Analysis. *Obesity Research & Clinical Practice*, 14(1), 1–8. https://doi.org/10.1016/j.orcp.2019.12.002

72. Lin, S., Cienfuegos, S., Ezpeleta, M., Gabel, K., Pavlou, V., Mulas, A., Chakos, K., McStay, M., Wu, J., Tussing-Humphreys, L., Alexandria, S. J., Sanchez, J., Unterman, T., & Varady, K. A. (2023). Time-Restricted Eating Without Calorie Counting for Weight Loss in a Racially Diverse Population: A Randomized Controlled Trial. *Annals of Internal Medicine*, 176(7), 885–95. https://doi.org/10.7326/M23-0052

73. Liu, D., Huang, Y., Huang, C., Yang, S., Wei, X., Zhang, P., Guo, D., Lin, J., Xu, B., Li, C., He, H., He, J., Liu, S., Shi, L., Xue, Y., & Zhang, H. (2022). Calorie Restriction With or Without Time-Restricted Eating in Weight Loss. *The New England Journal of Medicine*, 386(16), 1495–504. https://doi.org/10.1056/NEJMoa2114833

74. Maruthur, N. M., Pilla, S. J., White, K., Wu, B., Maw, M. T. T., Duan, D., Turkson-Ocran, R. A., Zhao, D., Charleston, J., Peterson, C. M., Dougherty, R. J., Schrack, J. A., Appel, L. J., Guallar, E., & Clark, J. M. (2024). Effect of Isocaloric, Time-Restricted Eating on Body Weight in Adults With Obesity: A Randomized Controlled Trial. *Annals of Internal Medicine*, 177(5), 549–58. https://doi.org/10.7326/M23-3132

75. Chen, J. H., Lu, L. W., Ge, Q., Feng, D., Yu, J., Liu, B., Zhang, R., Zhang, X., Ouyang, C., & Chen, F. (2023). Missing Puzzle Pieces of Time-Restricted-Eating (TRE) as a Long-Term Weight loss Strategy in Overweight and Obese People? A Systematic Review and Meta-Analysis of Randomized Controlled Trials. *Critical Reviews in Food Science and Nutrition*, 63(15), 2331–47. https://doi.org/10.1080/10408398.2021.1974335

76. Pellegrini, M., Cioffi, I., Evangelista, A., Ponzo, V., Goitre, I., Ciccone, G., Ghigo, E., & Bo, S. (2020). Effects of Time-Restricted Feeding on Body Weight and Metabolism. A Systematic Review and Meta-Analysis. *Reviews in Endocrine & Metabolic Disorders*, 21(1), 17–33. https://doi.org/10.1007/s11154-019-09524-w

77. Ezzati, A., Rosenkranz, S. K., Phelan, J., & Logan, C. (2023). The Effects of Isocaloric Intermittent Fasting vs Daily Caloric Restriction on Weight Loss and Metabolic Risk Factors for Noncommunicable Chronic Diseases: A Systematic Review of Randomized Controlled or Comparative Trials. *Journal of the Academy of Nutrition and Dietetics*, 123(2), 318–29.e1. https://doi.org/10.1016/j.jand.2022.09.013

78. Dalle Grave, R. (2020). Regular Eating, Not Intermittent Fasting, Is the Best Strategy for a Healthy Eating Control. *IJEDO*, 2, 5–7. https://doi.org/10.32044/ijedo.2020.02

79. Heilbronn, L. K., Smith, S. R., Martin, C. K., Anton, S. D., & Ravussin, E. (2005). Alternate-Day Fasting in Nonobese Subjects: Effects on Body Weight, Body Composition, and Energy Metabolism. *The American Journal of Clinical Nutrition*, 81(1), 69–73. https://doi.org/10.1093/ajcn/81.1.69

80. Ibid.

81. Varady, K. A., Bhutani, S., Church, E. C., & Klempel, M. C. (2009). Short-Term Modified Alternate-Day Fasting: A Novel Dietary Strategy for Weight Loss and Cardioprotection in Obese Adults. *The American Journal of Clinical Nutrition*, 90(5), 1138–43. https://doi.org/10.3945/ajcn.2009.28380

82. Eshghinia, S., & Mohammadzadeh, F. (2013). The Effects of Modified Alternate-Day Fasting Diet on Weight Loss and CAD Risk Factors in Overweight and Obese Women. *Journal of Diabetes and*

*Metabolic Disorders*, 12(1), 4. https://doi.org/10.1186/2251-6581-12-4

83. Heilbronn, L. K. et al. Alternate-Day Fasting in Nonobese Subjects.

84. Catenacci, V. A., Pan, Z., Ostendorf, D., Brannon, S., Gozansky, W. S., Mattson, M. P., Martin, B., MacLean, P. S., Melanson, E. L., & Troy Donahoo, W. (2016). A Randomized Pilot Study Comparing Zero-Calorie Alternate-Day Fasting to Daily Caloric Restriction in Adults With Obesity. *Obesity*, 24(9), 1874–83. https://doi.org/10.1002/oby.21581

85. Trepanowski, J. F., Kroeger, C. M., Barnosky, A., Klempel, M. C., Bhutani, S., Hoddy, K. K., Gabel, K., Freels, S., Rigdon, J., Rood, J., Ravussin, E., & Varady, K. A. (2017). Effect of Alternate-Day Fasting on Weight Loss, Weight Maintenance, and Cardioprotection Among Metabolically Healthy Obese Adults: A Randomized Clinical Trial. *JAMA Internal Medicine*, 177(7), 930–8. https://doi.org/10.1001/jamainternmed.2017.0936

86. Templeman, I., Smith, H. A., Chowdhury, E., Chen, Y. C., Carroll, H., Johnson-Bonson, D., Hengist, A., Smith, R., Creighton, J., Clayton, D., Varley, I., Karagounis, L. G., Wilhelmsen, A., Tsintzas, K., Reeves, S., Walhin, J. P., Gonzalez, J. T., Thompson, D., & Betts, J. A. (2021). A Randomized Controlled Trial to Isolate the Effects of Fasting and Energy Restriction on Weight Loss and Metabolic Health in Lean Adults. *Science Translational Medicine*, 13(598), eabd8034. https://doi.org/10.1126/scitranslmed.abd8034

87. Harvie, M. N., Pegington, M., Mattson, M. P., Frystyk, J., Dillon, B., Evans, G., Cuzick, J., Jebb, S. A., Martin, B., Cutler, R. G., Son, T. G., Maudsley, S., Carlson, O. D., Egan, J. M., Flyvbjerg, A., & Howell, A. (2011). The Effects of Intermittent or Continuous Energy Restriction on Weight Loss and Metabolic Disease Risk Markers: A Randomized Trial in Young Overweight Women. *International Journal of Obesity*, 35(5), 714–27. https://doi.org/10.1038/ijo.2010.171

88. Conley, M., Le Fevre, L., Haywood, C., & Proietto, J. (2018). Is Two Days of Intermittent Energy Restriction per Week a Feasible Weight Loss Approach in Obese Males? A Randomised Pilot Study. *Nutrition & Dietetics: The Journal of the Dietitians Association of Australia*, 75(1), 65–72. https://doi.org/10.1111/1747-0080.12372

89. Headland, M. L., Clifton, P. M., & Keogh, J. B. (2019). Effect of Intermittent Compared to Continuous Energy Restriction on Weight Loss and Weight Maintenance After 12 Months in Healthy Overweight or Obese Adults. *International Journal of Obesity*, 43(10),

2028–36. https://doi.org/10.1038/s41366-018-0247-2

90. Pinto, A. M., Bordoli, C., Buckner, L. P., Kim, C., Kaplan, P. C., Del Arenal, I. M., Jeffcock, E. J., & Hall, W. L. (2020). Intermittent Energy Restriction Is Comparable to Continuous Energy Restriction for Cardiometabolic Health in Adults With Central Obesity: A Randomized Controlled Trial; the Met-IER Study. *Clinical Nutrition*, 39(6), 1753–63. https://doi.org/10.1016/j.clnu.2019.07.014

91. Harvie, M. N. et al. The Effects of Intermittent or Continuous Energy Restriction on Weight Loss and Metabolic Disease Risk Markers.

92. Cook, F., Langdon-Daly, J., & Serpell, L. (2022). Compliance of Participants Undergoing a "5–2" Intermittent Fasting Diet and Impact on Body Weight. *Clinical Nutrition ESPEN*, 52, 257–61. https://doi.org/10.1016/j.clnesp.2022.08.012

93. Elortegui Pascual, P. et al. A Meta-Analysis Comparing the Effectiveness of Alternate Day Fasting, the 5:2 Diet, and Time-Restricted Eating for Weight Loss.

94. Gu, L., Fu, R., Hong, J., Ni, H., Yu, K., & Lou, H. (2022). Effects of Intermittent Fasting in Human Compared to a Non-intervention Diet and Caloric Restriction: A Meta-Analysis of Randomized Controlled Trials. *Frontiers in Nutrition*, 9, 871682. https://doi.org/10.3389/fnut.2022.871682

95. Schroor, M. M., Joris, P. J., Plat, J., & Mensink, R. P. (2024). Effects of Intermittent Energy Restriction Compared With Those of Continuous Energy Restriction on Body Composition and Cardiometabolic Risk Markers—A Systematic Review and Meta-Analysis of Randomized Controlled Trials in Adults. *Advances in Nutrition*, 15(1), 100130. https://doi.org/10.1016/j.advnut.2023.10.003

96. Vizthum, D., Katz, S. E., & Pacanowski, C. R. (2023). The Impact of Time Restricted Eating on Appetite and Disordered Eating in Adults: A Mixed Methods Systematic Review. *Appetite*, 183, 106452. https://doi.org/10.1016/j.appet.2023.106452

97. Stice, E., Davis, K., Miller, N. P., & Marti, C. N. (2008). Fasting Increases Risk for Onset of Binge Eating and Bulimic Pathology: A 5-Year Prospective Study. *Journal of Abnormal Psychology*, 117(4), 941–6. https://doi.org/10.1037/a0013644

98. Cuccolo, K., Kramer, R., Petros, T., & Thoennes, M. (2022). Intermittent Fasting Implementation and Association With Eating Disorder Symptomatology. *Eating Disorders*, 30(5), 471–91. https://doi.org/10.1080/10640266.2021.1922145

99. Schueler, J., Philip, S. R., Vitus, D., Engler, S., & Fields, S. A.

(2023). Group Differences in Binge Eating, Impulsivity, and Intuitive and Mindful Eating Among Intermittent Fasters and Non-fasters. *Appetite*, 182, 106416. https://doi.org/10.1016/j.appet.2022.106416

100. Blumberg, J., Hahn, S. L., & Bakke, J. (2023). Intermittent Fasting: Consider the Risks of Disordered Eating for Your Patient. *Clinical Diabetes and Endocrinology*, 9(1), 4. https://doi.org/10.1186/s40842-023-00152-7

101. Ibid.

102. Rickman, A. D., Williamson, D. A., Martin, C. K., Gilhooly, C. H., Stein, R. I., Bales, C. W., Roberts, S., & Das, S. K. (2011). The CALERIE Study: Design and Methods of an Innovative 25% Caloric Restriction Intervention. *Contemporary Clinical Trials*, 32(6), 874–81. https://doi.org/10.1016/j.cct.2011.07.002

103. Kraus, W. E., Bhapkar, M., Huffman, K. M., Pieper, C. F., Krupa Das, S., Redman, L. M., Villareal, D. T., Rochon, J., Roberts, S. B., Ravussin, E., Holloszy, J. O., Fontana, L., & CALERIE Investigators (2019). 2 Years of Calorie Restriction and Cardiometabolic Risk (CALERIE): Exploratory Outcomes of a Multicentre, Phase 2, Randomised Controlled Trial. *The Lancet: Diabetes & Endocrinology*, 7(9), 673–83.

https://doi.org/10.1016/S2213-8587(19)30151-2

104. Dorling, J. L., van Vliet, S., Huffman, K. M., Kraus, W. E., Bhapkar, M., Pieper, C. F., Stewart, T., Das, S. K., Racette, S. B., Roberts, S. B., Ravussin, E., Redman, L. M., Martin, C. K., & CALERIE Study Group (2021). Effects of Caloric Restriction on Human Physiological, Psychological, and Behavioral Outcomes: Highlights From CALERIE Phase 2. *Nutrition Reviews*, 79(1), 98–113. https://doi.org/10.1093/nutrit/nuaa085

105. Kraus, W. E. et al. 2 Years of Calorie Restriction and Cardiometabolic Risk (CALERIE).

## Chapter 4

1. Santos, I., et al. Prevalence of Personal Weight Control Attempts in Adults: A Systematic Review and Meta-Analysis.

2. Wadden, T. A., & Foster, G. D. (2006). Weight and Lifestyle Inventory (WALI). *Obesity*, 14 Suppl 2, 99–118S. https://doi.org/10.1038/oby.2006.289

3. Garaulet, M., Canteras, M., Morales, E., López-Guimera, G., Sánchez-Carracedo, D., & Corbalán-Tutau, M. D. (2012). Validation of a Questionnaire on Emotional Eating for Use in Cases of Obesity: The Emotional Eater Questionnaire (EEQ). *Nutricion Hospitalaria*, 27(2),

645–51. https://doi.org/10.1590/
S0212-16112012000200043

4. Craig, C. L., Marshall, A. L.,
Sjöström, M., Bauman, A. E.,
Booth, M. L., Ainsworth,
B. E., Pratt, M., Ekelund, U.,
Yngve, A., Sallis, J. F., & Oja, P.
(2003). International Physical
Activity Questionnaire:
12-Country Reliability and
Validity. *Medicine and Science
in Sports and Exercise*, 35(8),
1381–95. https://doi.org/10.1249/01.
MSS.0000078924.61453.FB

5. Lee, P. H., Macfarlane, D. J., Lam,
T. H., & Stewart, S. M. (2011).
Validity of the International
Physical Activity Questionnaire
Short Form (IPAQ-SF):
A Systematic Review. *The
International Journal of Behavioral
Nutrition and Physical Activity*,
8, 115. https://doi.org/10.1186/
1479-5868-8-115

6. Ravelli, M. N., & Schoeller, D. A.
(2020). Traditional Self-Reported
Dietary Instruments Are Prone to
Inaccuracies and New Approaches
Are Needed. *Frontiers in Nutrition*,
7, 90. https://doi.org/10.3389/
fnut.2020.00090

7. Wehling, H., & Lusher, J. (2019).
People With a Body Mass Index
≥30 Under-Report Their Dietary
Intake: A Systematic Review.
*Journal of Health Psychology*,
24(14), 2042–59. https://doi.
org/10.1177/1359105317714318

8. Fuente González, C. E., Chávez-
Servín, J. L., de la Torre-Carbot, K.,

Ronquillo González, D., Aguilera
Barreiro, M. L. Á., & Ojeda
Navarro, L. R. (2022). Relationship
Between Emotional Eating,
Consumption of Hyperpalatable
Energy-Dense Foods, and
Indicators of Nutritional Status:
A Systematic Review. *Journal of
Obesity*, 2022, 4243868. https://doi.
org/10.1155/2022/4243868

9. Dakanalis, A., et al. The
Association of Emotional Eating
With Overweight/Obesity,
Depression, Anxiety/Stress,
and Dietary Patterns.

10. Braden, A., Flatt, S. W., Boutelle,
K. N., Strong, D., Sherwood, N. E.,
& Rock, C. L. (2016). Emotional
Eating Is Associated With
Weight Loss Success Among
Adults Enrolled in a Weight Loss
Program. *Journal of Behavioral
Medicine*, 39(4), 727–32. https://doi.
org/10.1007/s10865-016-9728-8

11. Sainsbury, K., Evans, E. H.,
Pedersen, S., Marques, M. M.,
Teixeira, P. J., Lähteenmäki, L.,
Stubbs, R. J., Heitmann, B. L., &
Sniehotta, F. F. (2019). Attribution
of Weight Regain to Emotional
Reasons Amongst European
Adults With Overweight and
Obesity Who Regained Weight
Following a Weight Loss Attempt.
*Eating and Weight Disorders—
Studies on Anorexia, Bulimia, and
Obesity*, 24(2), 351–61. https://doi.
org/10.1007/s40519-018-0487-0

12. Ibid.

13. Wren, G. M., Koutoukidis, D. A., Scragg, J., Whitman, M., & Jebb, S. (2023). The Association Between Goal Setting and Weight Loss: Prospective Analysis of a Community Weight Loss Program. *Journal of Medical Internet Research*, 25, e43869. https://doi.org/10.2196/43869

14. Linde, J. A., Jeffery, R. W., Finch, E. A., Ng, D. M., & Rothman, A. J. (2004). Are Unrealistic Weight Loss Goals Associated With Outcomes for Overweight Women?. *Obesity Research*, 12(3), 569–76. https://doi.org/10.1038/oby.2004.65

15. Fabricatore, A. N., Wadden, T. A., Womble, L. G., Sarwer, D. B., Berkowitz, R. I., Foster, G. D., & Brock, J. R. (2007). The Role of Patients' Expectations and Goals in the Behavioral and Pharmacological Treatment of Obesity. *International Journal of Obesity* (2005), 31(11), 1739–45. https://doi.org/10.1038/sj.ijo.0803649

16. Foster, G. D., et al. What Is a Reasonable Weight Loss? Patients' Expectations and Evaluations of Obesity Treatment Outcomes.

17. Durant, N. H., Joseph, R. P., Affuso, O. H., Dutton, G. R., Robertson, H. T., & Allison, D. B. (2013). Empirical Evidence Does Not Support an Association Between Less Ambitious Pre-treatment Goals and Better Treatment Outcomes: A Meta-Analysis.

*Obesity Reviews: An Official Journal of the International Association for the Study of Obesity*, 14(7), 532–40. https://doi.org/10.1111/obr.12038

18. Foster, G. D., et al. What Is a Reasonable Weight Loss? Patients' Expectations and Evaluations of Obesity Treatment Outcomes.

19. Serrat, O. (2017). The Five Whys Technique. In: *Knowledge Solutions*. Springer, Singapore. https://doi.org/10.1007/978-981-10-0983-9_32

20. Teixeira, P. J., Carraça, E. V., Markland, D., Silva, M. N., & Ryan, R. M. (2012). Exercise, Physical Activity, and Self-Determination Theory: A Systematic Review. *The International Journal of Behavioral Nutrition and Physical Activity*, 9, 78. https://doi.org/10.1186/1479-5868-9-78

21. Panão, I., & Carraça, E. V. (2020). Effects of Exercise Motivations on Body Image and Eating Habits/Behaviours: A Systematic Review. *Nutrition & Dietetics: The Journal of the Dietitians Association of Australia*, 77(1), 41–59. https://doi.org/10.1111/1747-0080.12575

22. DiLillo, V., Siegfried, N. J., & West, D. S. (2003). Incorporating Motivational Interviewing Into Behavioral Obesity Treatment. *Cognitive and Behavioral Practice*, 10(2), 120–30. https://doi.org/10.1016/S1077-7229(03)80020-2

23. DiLillo, V., & West, D. S. (2011). Motivational Interviewing for

Weight Loss. *The Psychiatric Clinics of North America*, 34(4), 861–9. https://doi.org/10.1016/j.psc.2011.08.003

24. Cole, S. A., Sannidhi, D., Jadotte, Y. T., & Rozanski, A. (2023). Using Motivational Interviewing and Brief Action Planning for Adopting and Maintaining Positive Health Behaviors. *Progress in Cardiovascular Diseases*, 77, 86–94. https://doi.org/10.1016/j.pcad.2023.02.003

25. Barrett, S., Begg, S., O'Halloran, P., & Kingsley, M. (2018). Integrated Motivational Interviewing and Cognitive Behaviour Therapy for Lifestyle Mediators of Overweight and Obesity in Community-Dwelling Adults: A Systematic Review and Meta-Analyses. *BMC Public Health*, 18(1), 1160. https://doi.org/10.1186/s12889-018-6062-9

26. Morisano, D., Hirsh, J. B., Peterson, J. B., Pihl, R. O., & Shore, B. M. (2010). Setting, Elaborating, and Reflecting on Personal Goals Improves Academic Performance. *The Journal of Applied Psychology*, 95(2), 255–64. https://doi.org/10.1037/a0018478

27. Schippers, M. C., Morisano, D., Locke, E. A., Scheepers, A. W., Latham, G. P., & De Jong, E. M. (2020). Writing About Personal Goals and Plans Regardless of Goal Type Boosts Academic Performance. *Contemporary Educational Psychology*, 60,

101823. https://doi.org/10.1016/j.cedpsych.2019.101823

28. Morisano, D. et al. Setting, Elaborating, and Reflecting on Personal Goals Improves Academic Performance.

29. Epton, T., Currie, S., & Armitage, C. J. (2017). Unique Effects of Setting Goals on Behavior Change: Systematic Review and Meta-Analysis. *Journal of Consulting and Clinical Psychology*, 85(12), 1182–98. https://doi.org/10.1037/ccp0000260

30. Pearson, E. S. (2012). Goal Setting as a Health Behavior Change Strategy in Overweight and Obese Adults: A Systematic Literature Review Examining Intervention Components. *Patient Education and Counseling*, 87(1), 32–42. https://doi.org/10.1016/j.pec.2011.07.018

## Chapter 5

1. Garcia-Hermoso, A., López-Gil, J. F., Ramírez-Vélez, R., Alonso-Martínez, A. M., Izquierdo, M., & Ezzatvar, Y. (2023). Adherence to Aerobic and Muscle-Strengthening Activities Guidelines: A Systematic Review and Meta-Analysis of 3.3 Million Participants Across 32 Countries. *British Journal of Sports Medicine*, 57(4), 225–9. https://doi.org/10.1136/bjsports-2022-106189

2. Guthold, R., Stevens, G. A., Riley, L. M., & Bull, F. C. (2018). Worldwide Trends in Insufficient Physical Activity From 2001

to 2016: A Pooled Analysis of 358 Population-Based Surveys With 1·9 Million Participants. *The Lancet. Global Health*, 6(10), e1077–86. https://doi.org/10.1016/S2214-109X(18)30357-7

3. Grannell, A., Fallon, F., Al-Najim, W., & Le Roux, C. (2021). Obesity and Responsibility: Is It Time to Rethink Agency? *Obesity Reviews: An Official Journal of the International Association for the Study of Obesity*, 22(8), e13270. https://doi.org/10.1111/obr.13270

4. Jebb, S. A., & Aveyard, P. (2023). "Willpower" Is Not Enough: Time for a New Approach to Public Health Policy to Prevent Obesity. *BMC Medicine*, 21(1), 89. https://doi.org/10.1186/s12916-023-02803-z

5. Ainslie G. (2020). Willpower With and Without Effort. *Behavioral and Brain Sciences*, 44, e30. https://doi.org/10.1017/S0140525X20000357

6. Mischel, W., Ayduk, O., Berman, M. G., Casey, B. J., Gotlib, I. H., Jonides, J., Kross, E., Teslovich, T., Wilson, N. L., Zayas, V., & Shoda, Y. (2011). "Willpower" Over the Life Span: Decomposing Self-Regulation. *Social Cognitive and Affective Neuroscience*, 6(2), 252–6. https://doi.org/10.1093/scan/nsq081

7. Duckworth, A. L., Milkman, K. L., & Laibson, D. (2018). Beyond Willpower: Strategies for Reducing Failures of Self-Control. *Psychological Science in the Public Interest: A Journal of the American Psychological Society*, 19(3), 102–29. https://doi.org/10.1177/1529100618821893

8. James, W. (1890). *The Principles of Psychology*, Vol. 1. Henry Holt and Co. https://doi.org/10.1037/10538–000

9. Van't Riet, J., Sijtsema, S. J., Dagevos, H., & De Bruijn, G. J. (2011). The Importance of Habits in Eating Behaviour. An Overview and Recommendations for Future Research. *Appetite*, 57(3), 585–96. https://doi.org/10.1016/j.appet.2011.07.010

10. Gardner, B., Rebar, A. L., & Lally, P. (2020). Habit Interventions. In: *The Handbook of Behaviour Change*. Cambridge University Press, 599–616. https://doi.org/10.1017/9781108677318.041

11. Ibid.

12. Gardner, B., Lally, P., & Wardle, J. (2012). Making Health Habitual: The Psychology of "Habit-Formation" and General Practice. *The British Journal of General Practice: The Journal of the Royal College of General Practitioners*, 62(605), 664–6. https://doi.org/10.3399/bjgp12X659466

13. Lally, P., Chipperfield, A., & Wardle, J. (2008). Healthy Habits: Efficacy of Simple Advice on Weight Control Based on a Habit-Formation Model. *International Journal of Obesity*, 32(4), 700–707. https://doi.org/10.1038/sj.ijo.0803771

14. Cleo, G., Glasziou, P., Beller, E., Isenring, E., & Thomas, R. (2019). Habit-Based Interventions for Weight Loss Maintenance in Adults With Overweight and Obesity: A Randomized Controlled Trial. *International Journal of Obesity*, 43(2), 374–83. https://doi.org/10.1038/s41366-018-0067-4

15. Cleo, G., Isenring, E., Thomas, R., & Glasziou, P. (2017). Could Habits Hold the Key to Weight Loss Maintenance? A Narrative Review. *Journal of Human Nutrition and Dietetics: The Official Journal of the British Dietetic Association*, 30(5), 655–64. https://doi.org/10.1111/jhn.12456

16. Cleo, G., Beller, E., Glasziou, P., Isenring, E., & Thomas, R. (2020). Efficacy of Habit-Based Weight Loss Interventions: A Systematic Review and Meta-Analysis. *Journal of Behavioral Medicine*, 43(4), 519–32. https://doi.org/10.1007/s10865-019-00100-w

17. Robinson, E., Khuttan, M., McFarland-Lesser, I., Patel, Z., & Jones, A. (2022). Calorie Reformulation: A Systematic Review and Meta-Analysis Examining the Effect of Manipulating Food Energy Density on Daily Energy Intake. *The International Journal of Behavioral Nutrition and Physical Activity*, 19(1), 48. https://doi.org/10.1186/s12966-022-01287-z

18. Klos, B., Cook, J., Crepaz, L., Weiland, A., Zipfel, S., & Mack, I. (2023). Impact of Energy Density on Energy Intake in Children and Adults: A Systematic Review and Meta-Analysis of Randomized Controlled Trials. *European Journal of Nutrition*, 62(3), 1059–76. https://doi.org/10.1007/s00394-022-03054-z

19. Stewart, T. M., Martin, C. K., & Williamson, D. A. (2022). The Complicated Relationship Between Dieting, Dietary Restraint, Caloric Restriction, and Eating Disorders: Is a Shift in Public Health Messaging Warranted?. *International Journal of Environmental Research and Public Health*, 19(1), 491. https://doi.org/10.3390/ijerph19010491

20. Dakin, C., Beaulieu, K., Hopkins, M., Gibbons, C., Finlayson, G., & Stubbs, R. J. (2023). Do Eating Behavior Traits Predict Energy Intake and Body Mass Index? A Systematic Review and Meta-Analysis. *Obesity Reviews: An Official Journal of the International Association for the Study of Obesity*, 24(1), e13515. https://doi.org/10.1111/obr.13515

21. Lee, S. H., Moore, L. V., Park, S., Harris, D. M., & Blanck, H. M. (2022). Adults Meeting Fruit and Vegetable Intake Recommendations—United States, 2019. MMWR. *Morbidity and Mortality Weekly Report*, 71(1), 1–9. https://doi.org/10.15585/mmwr.mm7101a1

22. Wallace, T. C., Bailey, R. L., Blumberg, J. B., Burton-Freeman, B., Chen, C. O., Crowe-White, K. M., Drewnowski, A., Hooshmand, S., Johnson, E., Lewis, R., Murray, R., Shapses, S. A., & Wang, D. D. (2020). Fruits, Vegetables, and Health: A Comprehensive Narrative, Umbrella Review of the Science and Recommendations for Enhanced Public Policy to Improve Intake. *Critical Reviews in Food Science and Nutrition*, 60(13), 2174–211. https://doi.org/10.1080/10408398.2019.1632258

23. Wang, D. D., Li, Y., Bhupathiraju, S. N., Rosner, B. A., Sun, Q., Giovannucci, E. L., Rimm, E. B., Manson, J. E., Willett, W. C., Stampfer, M. J., & Hu, F. B. (2021). Fruit and Vegetable Intake and Mortality: Results From 2 Prospective Cohort Studies of US Men and Women and a Meta-Analysis of 26 Cohort Studies. *Circulation*, 143(17), 1642–54. https://doi.org/10.1161/circulationaha.120.048996

24. Ello-Martin, J. A., Roe, L. S., Ledikwe, J. H., Beach, A. M., & Rolls, B. J. (2007). Dietary Energy Density in the Treatment of Obesity: A Year-Long Trial Comparing 2 Weight loss Diets. *The American Journal of Clinical Nutrition*, 85(6), 1465–77. https://doi.org/10.1093/ajcn/85.6.1465

25. Rolls, B. J., Roe, L. S., & Meengs, J. S. (2010). Portion Size Can Be Used Strategically to Increase Vegetable Consumption in Adults. *The American Journal of Clinical Nutrition*, 91(4), 913–22. https://doi.org/10.3945/ajcn.2009.28801

26. Blatt, A. D., Roe, L. S., & Rolls, B. J. (2011). Hidden Vegetables: An Effective Strategy to Reduce Energy Intake and Increase Vegetable Intake in Adults. *The American Journal of Clinical Nutrition*, 93(4), 756–63. https://doi.org/10.3945/ajcn.110.009332

27. Spill, M. K., Birch, L. L., Roe, L. S., & Rolls, B. J. (2011). Hiding Vegetables to Reduce Energy Density: An Effective Strategy to Increase Children's Vegetable Intake and Reduce Energy Intake. *The American Journal of Clinical Nutrition*, 94(3), 735–41. https://doi.org/10.3945/ajcn.111.015206

28. Rolls, B. J., Roe, L. S., & Meengs, J. S. (2004). Salad and Satiety: Energy Density and Portion Size of a First-Course Salad Affect Energy Intake at Lunch. *Journal of the American Dietetic Association*, 104(10), 1570–6. https://doi.org/10.1016/j.jada.2004.07.001

29. Flood-Obbagy, J. E., & Rolls, B. J. (2009). The Effect of Fruit in Different Forms on Energy Intake and Satiety at a Meal. *Appetite*, 52(2), 416–22. https://doi.org/10.1016/j.appet.2008.12.001

30. Redden, J. P., Mann, T., Vickers, Z., Mykerezi, E., Reicks, M., & Elsbernd, S. (2015). Serving First in Isolation Increases Vegetable

Intake Among Elementary Schoolchildren. *PloS One*, 10(4), e0121283. https://doi.org/10.1371/journal.pone.0121283

31. Elsbernd, S. L., Reicks, M. M., Mann, T. L., Redden, J. P., Mykerezi, E., & Vickers, Z. M. (2016). Serving Vegetables First: A Strategy to Increase Vegetable Consumption in Elementary School Cafeterias. *Appetite*, 96, 111–15. https://doi.org/10.1016/j.appet.2015.09.001

32. Livingstone, K. M., Burton, M., Brown, A. K., & McNaughton, S. A. (2020). Exploring Barriers to Meeting Recommendations for Fruit and Vegetable Intake Among Adults in Regional Areas: A Mixed-Methods Analysis of Variations Across Socio-Demographics. *Appetite*, 153, 104750. https://doi.org/10.1016/j.appet.2020.104750

33. Li, L., Pegg, R. B., Eitenmiller, R. R., Chun, J. Y., & Kerrihard, A. L. (2017). Selected Nutrient Analyses of Fresh, Fresh-Stored, and Frozen Fruits and Vegetables. *Journal of Food Composition and Analysis*, 59, 8–17. https://doi.org/10.1016/j.jfca.2017.02.002

34. Rickman, J. C., Barrett, D. M., & Bruhn, C. M. (2007). Nutritional Comparison of Fresh, Frozen and Canned Fruits and Vegetables. Part 1. Vitamins C and B and Phenolic Compounds. *Journal of the Science of Food and Agriculture*, 87(6), 930–44. https://doi.org/10.1002/jsfa.2825

35. Freedman, M. R., & Fulgoni, V. L., III (2016). Canned Vegetable and Fruit Consumption Is Associated With Changes in Nutrient Intake and Higher Diet Quality in Children and Adults: National Health and Nutrition Examination Survey 2001–2010. *Journal of the Academy of Nutrition and Dietetics*, 116(6), 940–8. https://doi.org/10.1016/j.jand.2015.10.013

36. Wang, D. D. et al. Fruit and Vegetable Intake and Mortality.

37. US Department of Agriculture and US Department of Health and Human Services (2020). Dietary Guidelines for Americans, 2020–2025, 9th Edition. Retrieved from https://www.dietaryguidelines.gov/sites/default/files/2020-12/Dietary_Guidelines_for_Americans_2020-2025.pdf

38. Public Health England (2019). Saturated Fats and Health: SACN Report. Retrieved from https://www.gov.uk/government/publications/saturated-fats-and-health-sacn-report

39. Peterson, S., Sigman-Grant, M., Eissenstat, B., & Kris-Etherton, P. (1999). Impact of Adopting Lower-Fat Food Choices on Energy and Nutrient Intakes of American Adults. *Journal of the American Dietetic Association*, 99(2), 177–83. https://doi.org/10.1016/S0002-8223(99)00043-7

40. Borela, V. L., De Alencar, E. R., Mendonça, M. A., Han, H., Raposo, A., Ariza-Montes, A.,

Araya-Castillo, L., & Zandonadi, R. P. (2022). Influence of Different Cooking Methods on Fillet Steak Physicochemical Characteristics. *International Journal of Environmental Research and Public Health*, 19(1), 606. https://doi.org/10.3390/ijerph19010606

41. Gerber, N., Scheeder, M. R., & Wenk, C. (2009). The Influence of Cooking and Fat Trimming on the Actual Nutrient Intake From Meat. *Meat Science*, 81(1), 148–54. https://doi.org/10.1016/j.meatsci.2008.07.012

42. Lally, P. et al. Healthy Habits: Efficacy of Simple Advice on Weight Control Based on a Habit-Formation Model.

43. Schwingshackl, L., Zähringer, J., Beyerbach, J., Werner, S. S., Heseker, H., Koletzko, B., & Meerpohl, J. J. (2021). Total Dietary Fat Intake, Fat Quality, and Health Outcomes: A Scoping Review of Systematic Reviews of Prospective Studies. *Annals of Nutrition & Metabolism*, 77(1), 4–15. https://doi.org/10.1159/000515058

44. Huang, C., Dumanovsky, T., Silver, L. D., Nonas, C., & Bassett, M. T. (2009). Calories From Beverages Purchased at 2 Major Coffee Chains in New York City, 2007. *Preventing Chronic Disease*, 6(4), A118.

45. Duffey, K. J., & Popkin, B. M. (2007). Shifts in Patterns and Consumption of Beverages Between 1965 and 2002. *Obesity*, 15(11), 2739–47. https://doi.org/10.1038/oby.2007.326

46. Pan, A., & Hu, F. B. (2011). Effects of Carbohydrates on Satiety: Differences Between Liquid and Solid Food. *Current Opinion in Clinical Nutrition and Metabolic Care*, 14(4), 385–90. https://doi.org/10.1097/MCO.0b013e328346df36

47. Appelhans, B. M., Bleil, M. E., Waring, M. E., Schneider, K. L., Nackers, L. M., Busch, A. M., Whited, M. C., & Pagoto, S. L. (2013). Beverages Contribute Extra Calories to Meals and Daily Energy Intake in Overweight and Obese Women. *Physiology & Behavior*, 122, 129–33. https://doi.org/10.1016/j.physbeh.2013.09.004

48. Tran, Q. D., Nguyen, T. H. H., Le, C. L., Hoang, L. V., Vu, T. Q. C., Phan, N. Q., & Bui, T. T. (2023). Sugar-Sweetened Beverages Consumption Increases the Risk of Metabolic Syndrome and Its Components in Adults: Consistent and Robust Evidence From an Umbrella Review. *Clinical Nutrition ESPEN*, 57, 655–64. https://doi.org/10.1016/j.clnesp.2023.08.001

49. Andreyeva, T., Marple, K., Marinello, S., Moore, T. E., & Powell, L. M. (2022). Outcomes Following Taxation of Sugar-Sweetened Beverages: A Systematic Review and Meta-Analysis. *JAMA Network Open*, 5(6), e2215276.

https://doi.org/10.1001/jamanetworkopen.2022.15276

50. Harrold, J. A., Hill, S., Radu, C., Thomas, P., Thorp, P., Hardman, C. A., Christiansen, P., & Halford, J. C. G. (2024). Non-nutritive Sweetened Beverages Versus Water After a 52-Week Weight Management Programme: A Randomised Controlled Trial. *International Journal of Obesity*, 48(1), 83–93. https://doi.org/10.1038/s41366-023-01393-3

51. McGlynn, N. D., Khan, T. A., Wang, L., Zhang, R., Chiavaroli, L., Au-Yeung, F., Lee, J. J., Noronha, J. C., Comelli, E. M., Blanco Mejia, S., Ahmed, A., Malik, V. S., Hill, J. O., Leiter, L. A., Agarwal, A., Jeppesen, P. B., Rahelic, D., Kahleová, H., Salas-Salvadó, J., Kendall, C. W. C.,…Sievenpiper, J. L. (2022). Association of Low- and No-Calorie Sweetened Beverages as a Replacement for Sugar-Sweetened Beverages With Body Weight and Cardiometabolic Risk: A Systematic Review and Meta-analysis. *JAMA Network Open*, 5(3), e222092. https://doi.org/10.1001/jamanetworkopen.2022.2092

52. Nguyen, M., Jarvis, S. E., Tinajero, M. G., Yu, J., Chiavaroli, L., Mejia, S. B., Khan, T. A., Tobias, D. K., Willett, W. C., Hu, F. B., Hanley, A. J., Birken, C. S., Sievenpiper, J. L., & Malik, V. S. (2023). Sugar-Sweetened Beverage Consumption and Weight Gain in Children and Adults: A Systematic Review and Meta-Analysis of Prospective Cohort Studies and Randomized Controlled Trials. *The American Journal of Clinical Nutrition*, 117(1), 160–74. https://doi.org/10.1016/j.ajcnut.2022.11.008

53. Tran, Q. D., et al. Sugar-Sweetened Beverages Consumption Increases the Risk of Metabolic Syndrome and Its Components in Adults: Consistent and Robust Evidence From an Umbrella Review.

54. Warburton, D. E. R., & Bredin, S. S. D. (2017). Health Benefits of Physical Activity: A Systematic Review of Current Systematic Reviews. *Current Opinion in Cardiology*, 32(5), 541–56. https://doi.org/10.1097/HCO.0000000000000437

55. Ramakrishnan, R., He, J. R., Ponsonby, A. L., Woodward, M., Rahimi, K., Blair, S. N., & Dwyer, T. (2021). Objectively Measured Physical Activity and All Cause Mortality: A Systematic Review and Meta-Analysis. *Preventive Medicine*, 143, 106356. https://doi.org/10.1016/j.ypmed.2020.106356

56. Yuan, Y., Lin, S., Lin, W., Huang, F., & Zhu, P. (2022). Modifiable Predictive Factors and All-Cause Mortality in the Non-hospitalized Elderly Population: An Umbrella Review of Meta-Analyses. *Experimental Gerontology*, 163, 111792. https://doi.org/10.1016/j.exger.2022.111792

57. Dale, L. P., Vanderloo, L., Moore, S., & Faulkner, G. (2019). Physical Activity and Depression, Anxiety, and Self-Esteem in Children and Youth: An Umbrella Systematic Review. *Mental Health and Physical Activity*, 16, 66–79. https://doi.org/10.1016/j.mhpa.2018.12.001

58. Noetel, M., Sanders, T., Gallardo-Gómez, D., Taylor, P., Del Pozo Cruz, B., van den Hoek, D., Smith, J. J., Mahoney, J., Spathis, J., Moresi, M., Pagano, R., Pagano, L., Vasconcellos, R., Arnott, H., Varley, B., Parker, P., Biddle, S., & Lonsdale, C. (2024). Effect of Exercise for Depression: Systematic Review and Network Meta-Analysis of Randomised Controlled Trials. *BMJ*, 384, e075847. https://doi.org/10.1136/bmj-2023-075847

59. Warburton, D. E. R., & Bredin, S. S. D., Health Benefits of Physical Activity: A Systematic Review of Current Systematic Reviews.

60. Ainsworth, B. E., Haskell, W. L., Herrmann, S. D., Meckes, N., Bassett, D. R., Jr., Tudor-Locke, C., Greer, J. L., Vezina, J., Whitt-Glover, M. C., & Leon, A. S. (2011). 2011 Compendium of Physical Activities: A Second Update of Codes and MET Values. *Medicine and Science in Sports and Exercise*, 43(8), 1575–81. https://doi.org/10.1249/MSS.0b013e31821ece12

61. Maclean, P. S., Bergouignan, A., Cornier, M. A., & Jackman, M. R. (2011). Biology's Response to Dieting: The Impetus for Weight Regain. *American Journal of Physiology: Regulatory, Integrative and Comparative Physiology*, 301(3), R581–600. https://doi.org/10.1152/ajpregu.00755.2010

62. Thorogood, A., Mottillo, S., Shimony, A., Filion, K. B., Joseph, L., Genest, J., Pilote, L., Poirier, P., Schiffrin, E. L., & Eisenberg, M. J. (2011). Isolated Aerobic Exercise and Weight Loss: A Systematic Review and Meta-Analysis of Randomized Controlled Trials. *The American Journal of Medicine*, 124(8), 747–55. https://doi.org/10.1016/j.amjmed.2011.02.037

63. Flack, K. D., Ufholz, K., Johnson, L., Fitzgerald, J. S., & Roemmich, J. N. (2018). Energy Compensation in Response to Aerobic Exercise Training in Overweight Adults. *American Journal of Physiology: Regulatory, Integrative and Comparative Physiology*, 315(4), R619–26. https://doi.org/10.1152/ajpregu.00071.2018

64. Martin, C. K., Johnson, W. D., Myers, C. A., Apolzan, J. W., Earnest, C. P., Thomas, D. M., Rood, J. C., Johannsen, N. M., Tudor-Locke, C., Harris, M., Hsia, D. S., & Church, T. S. (2019). Effect of Different Doses of Supervised Exercise on Food Intake, Metabolism, and Non-exercise Physical Activity: The E-Mechanic Randomized Controlled Trial. *The American Journal of Clinical*

*Nutrition*, 110(3), 583–92. https://doi.org/10.1093/ajcn/nqz054

65. Careau, V., Halsey, L. G., Pontzer, H., Ainslie, P. N., Andersen, L. F., Anderson, L. J., Arab, L., Baddou, I., Bedu-Addo, K., Blaak, E. E., Blanc, S., Bonomi, A. G., Bouten, C. V. C., Buchowski, M. S., Butte, N. F., Camps, S. G. J. A., Close, G. L., Cooper, J. A., Das, S. K., Cooper, R.,...I A E A DLW Database Group (2021). Energy Compensation and Adiposity in Humans. *Current Biology*, 31(20), 4659–66.e2. https://doi.org/10.1016/j.cub.2021.08.016

66. Fernández-Verdejo, R., Alcantara, J. M. A., Galgani, J. E., Acosta, F. M., Migueles, J. H., Amaro-Gahete, F. J., Labayen, I., Ortega, F. B., & Ruiz, J. R. (2021). Deciphering the Constrained Total Energy Expenditure Model in Humans by Associating Accelerometer-Measured Physical Activity From Wrist and Hip. *Scientific Reports*, 11(1), 12302. https://doi.org/10.1038/s41598-021-91750-x

67. Gonzalez, J. T., Batterham, A. M., Atkinson, G., & Thompson, D. (2023). Perspective: Is the Response of Human Energy Expenditure to Increased Physical Activity Additive or Constrained? *Advances in Nutrition*, 14(3), 406–19. https://doi.org/10.1016/j.advnut.2023.02.003

68. Thomas, D. M., Kyle, T. K., & Stanford, F. C. (2015). The Gap Between Expectations and Reality of Exercise-Induced Weight Loss Is Associated With Discouragement. *Preventive Medicine*, 81, 357–60. https://doi.org/10.1016/j.ypmed.2015.10.001

69. Recchia, F., Leung, C. K., Yu, A. P., Leung, W., Yu, D. J., Fong, D. Y., Montero, D., Lee, C. H., Wong, S. H. S., & Siu, P. M. (2023). Dose-Response Effects of Exercise and Caloric Restriction on Visceral Adiposity in Overweight and Obese Adults: A Systematic Review and Meta-Analysis of Randomised Controlled Trials. *British Journal of Sports Medicine*, 57(16), 1035–41. https://doi.org/10.1136/bjsports-2022-106304

70. Verheggen, R. J., Maessen, M. F., Green, D. J., Hermus, A. R., Hopman, M. T., & Thijssen, D. H. (2016). A Systematic Review and Meta-Analysis on the Effects of Exercise Training Versus Hypocaloric Diet: Distinct Effects on Body Weight and Visceral Adipose Tissue. *Obesity Reviews : An Official Journal of the International Association for the Study of Obesity*, 17(8), 664–90. https://doi.org/10.1111/obr.12406

71. Neeland, I. J., Ross, R., Després, J. P., Matsuzawa, Y., Yamashita, S., Shai, I., Seidell, J., Magni, P., Santos, R. D., Arsenault, B., Cuevas, A., Hu, F. B., Griffin, B., Zambon, A., Barter, P., Fruchart, J. C., Eckel, R. H., International Atherosclerosis Society, & International Chair

on Cardiometabolic Risk Working Group on Visceral Obesity (2019). Visceral and Ectopic Fat, Atherosclerosis, and Cardiometabolic Disease: A Position Statement. *The Lancet: Diabetes & Endocrinology*, 7(9), 715–25. https://doi.org/10.1016/S2213-8587(19)30084-1

72. Bellicha, A., van Baak, M. A., Battista, F., Beaulieu, K., Blundell, J. E., Busetto, L., Carraça, E. V., Dicker, D., Encantado, J., Ermolao, A., Farpour-Lambert, N., Pramono, A., Woodward, E., & Oppert, J. M. (2021). Effect of Exercise Training on Weight Loss, Body Composition Changes, and Weight Maintenance in Adults With Overweight or Obesity: An Overview of 12 Systematic Reviews and 149 Studies. *Obesity Reviews: An Official Journal of the International Association for the Study of Obesity*, 22 Suppl 4, e13256. https://doi.org/10.1111/obr.13256

73. Bull, F. C., Al-Ansari, S. S., Biddle, S., Borodulin, K., Buman, M. P., Cardon, G., Carty, C., Chaput, J. P., Chastin, S., Chou, R., Dempsey, P. C., DiPietro, L., Ekelund, U., Firth, J., Friedenreich, C. M., Garcia, L., Gichu, M., Jago, R., Katzmarzyk, P. T., Lambert, E.,...Willumsen, J. F. (2020). World Health Organization 2020 Guidelines on Physical Activity and Sedentary Behaviour. *British Journal of Sports Medicine*, 54(24), 1451–62. https://doi.org/10.1136/bjsports-2020-102955

74. McCrady-Spitzer, S. K., & Levine, J. A. (2012). Nonexercise Activity Thermogenesis: A Way Forward to Treat the Worldwide Obesity Epidemic. *Surgery for Obesity and Related Diseases: Official Journal of the American Society for Bariatric Surgery*, 8(5), 501–6. https://doi.org/10.1016/j.soard.2012.08.001

75. Malaeb, S., Perez-Leighton, C. E., Noble, E. E., & Billington, C. (2019). A "NEAT" Approach to Obesity Prevention in the Modern Work Environment. *Workplace Health & Safety*, 67(3), 102–10. https://doi.org/10.1177/2165079918790980

76. Rizzato, A., et al. Non-exercise Activity Thermogenesis in the Workplace: The Office Is on Fire.

77. Villablanca, P. A., et al. Nonexercise Activity Thermogenesis in Obesity Management.

78. Ibid.

79. Schneider, P. L., Bassett, D. R., Jr., Thompson, D. L., Pronk, N. P., & Bielak, K. M. (2006). Effects of a 10,000 Steps per Day Goal in Overweight Adults. *American Journal of Health Promotion*, 21(2), 85–9. https://doi.org/10.4278/0890-1171-21.2.85

80. Musto, A., Jacobs, K., Nash, M., DelRossi, G., & Perry, A. (2010). The Effects of an Incremental Approach to 10,000 Steps/Day on Metabolic Syndrome Components

in Sedentary Overweight Women. *Journal of Physical Activity & Health*, 7(6), 737–45. https://doi.org/10.1123/jpah.7.6.737

81. Saint-Maurice, P. F., Troiano, R. P., Bassett, D. R., Jr., Graubard, B. I., Carlson, S. A., Shiroma, E. J., Fulton, J. E., & Matthews, C. E. (2020). Association of Daily Step Count and Step Intensity With Mortality Among US Adults. *JAMA*, 323(12), 1151–60. https://doi.org/10.1001/jama.2020.1382

82. Sheng, M., Yang, J., Bao, M., Chen, T., Cai, R., Zhang, N., Chen, H., Liu, M., Wu, X., Zhang, B., Liu, Y., & Chao, J. (2021). The Relationships Between Step Count and All-Cause Mortality and Cardiovascular Events: A Dose-Response Meta-Analysis. *Journal of Sport and Health Science*, 10(6), 620–28. https://doi.org/10.1016/j.jshs.2021.09.004

83. Ibid.

84. Islam, H., Gibala, M. J., & Little, J. P. (2022). Exercise Snacks: A Novel Strategy to Improve Cardiometabolic Health. *Exercise and Sport Sciences Reviews*, 50(1), 31–7. https://doi.org/10.1249/JES.0000000000000275

85. Sanders, J. P., Biddle, S. J. H., Gokal, K., Sherar, L. B., Skrybant, M., Parretti, H. M., Ives, N., Yates, T., Mutrie, N., Daley, A. J., & Snacktivity Study Team (2021). "Snacktivity™" to Increase Physical Activity: Time to Try Something Different?

*Preventive Medicine*, 153, 106851. https://doi.org/10.1016/j.ypmed.2021.106851

86. Jones, M. D., Clifford, B. K., Stamatakis, E., & Gibbs, M. T. (2024). Exercise Snacks and Other Forms of Intermittent Physical Activity for Improving Health in Adults and Older Adults: A Scoping Review of Epidemiological, Experimental and Qualitative Studies. *Sports Medicine*, 54, 813–35. https://doi.org/10.1007/s40279-023-01983-1

87. Han, M., Qie, R., Shi, X., Yang, Y., Lu, J., Hu, F., Zhang, M., Zhang, Z., Hu, D., & Zhao, Y. (2022). Cardiorespiratory Fitness and Mortality From All Causes, Cardiovascular Disease and Cancer: Dose-Response Meta-Analysis of Cohort Studies. *British Journal of Sports Medicine*, 56(13), 733–9. https://doi.org/10.1136/bjsports-2021-104876

88. Lally, P. et al. Healthy Habits: Efficacy of Simple Advice on Weight Control Based on a Habit-Formation Model.

89. Li, J., Cao, D., Huang, Y., Chen, Z., Wang, R., Dong, Q.,…& Liu, L. (2022). Sleep Duration and Health Outcomes: An Umbrella Review. *Sleep and Breathing*, 26, 1479–501. https://doi.org/10.1007/s11325-021-02458-1

90. Mosavat, M., Mirsanjari, M., Arabiat, D., Smyth, A., & Whitehead, L. (2021). The Role of Sleep Curtailment on

Leptin Levels in Obesity and Diabetes Mellitus. *Obesity Facts*, 14(2), 214–21. https://doi.org/10.1159/000514095

91. Schmid, S. M., Hallschmid, M., Jauch-Chara, K., Born, J., & Schultes, B. (2008). A Single Night of Sleep Deprivation Increases Ghrelin Levels and Feelings of Hunger in Normal-Weight Healthy Men. *Journal of Sleep Research*, 17(3), 331–4. https://doi.org/10.1111/j.1365-2869.2008.00662.x

92. van Egmond, L. T., Meth, E. M. S., Engström, J., Ilemosoglou, M., Keller, J. A., Vogel, H., & Benedict, C. (2023). Effects of Acute Sleep Loss on Leptin, Ghrelin, and Adiponectin in Adults With Healthy Weight and Obesity: A Laboratory Study. *Obesity*, 31(3), 635–41. https://doi.org/10.1002/oby.23616

93. Brondel, L., Romer, M. A., Nougues, P. M., Touyarou, P., & Davenne, D. (2010). Acute Partial Sleep Deprivation Increases Food Intake in Healthy Men. *The American Journal of Clinical Nutrition*, 91(6), 1550–9. https://doi.org/10.3945/ajcn.2009.28523

94. Nedeltcheva, A. V., Kilkus, J. M., Imperial, J., Kasza, K., Schoeller, D. A., & Penev, P. D. (2009). Sleep Curtailment Is Accompanied by Increased Intake of Calories From Snacks. *The American Journal of Clinical Nutrition*, 89(1),

126–33. https://doi.org/10.3945/ajcn.2008.26574

95. Brondel, L. et al. Acute Partial Sleep Deprivation Increases Food Intake in Healthy Men.

96. Nedeltcheva, A. V., Kilkus, J. M., Imperial, J., Schoeller, D. A., & Penev, P. D. (2010). Insufficient Sleep Undermines Dietary Efforts to Reduce Adiposity. *Annals of Internal Medicine*, 153(7), 435–41. https://doi.org/10.7326/0003-4819-153-7-201010050-00006

97. Tasali, E., Wroblewski, K., Kahn, E., Kilkus, J., & Schoeller, D. A. (2022). Effect of Sleep Extension on Objectively Assessed Energy Intake Among Adults With Overweight in Real-Life Settings: A Randomized Clinical Trial. *JAMA Internal Medicine*, 182(4), 365–74. https://doi.org/10.1001/jamainternmed.2021.8098

98. Ibid.

99. Jåbekk, P., Jensen, R. M., Sandell, M. B., Haugen, E., Katralen, L. M., & Bjorvatn, B. (2020). A Randomized Controlled Pilot Trial of Sleep Health Education on Body Composition Changes Following 10 Weeks' Resistance Exercise. *The Journal of Sports Medicine and Physical Fitness*, 60(5), 743–8. https://doi.org/10.23736/S0022-4707.20.10136-1

100. Ibid.

101. Kohanmoo, A., et al. Effect of Short- and Long-Term Protein Consumption on Appetite

and Appetite-Regulating Gastrointestinal Hormones, a Systematic Review and Meta-Analysis of Randomized Controlled Trials.

102. Ludwig, D. S., Majzoub, J. A., Al-Zahrani, A., Dallal, G. E., Blanco, I., & Roberts, S. B. (1999). High Glycemic Index Foods, Overeating, and Obesity. *Pediatrics*, 103(3), E26. https://doi.org/10.1542/peds.103.3.e26

103. Vander Wal, J. S., Gupta, A., Khosla, P., & Dhurandhar, N. V. (2008). Egg Breakfast Enhances Weight Loss. *International Journal of Obesity*, 32(10), 1545–51. https://doi.org/10.1038/ijo.2008.130

104. Leidy, H. J., Hoertel, H. A., Douglas, S. M., Higgins, K. A., & Shafer, R. S. (2015). A High-Protein Breakfast Prevents Body Fat Gain, Through Reductions in Daily Intake and Hunger, in "Breakfast Skipping" Adolescents. *Obesity*, 23(9), 1761–4. https://doi.org/10.1002/oby.21185

105. Qiu, M., Zhang, Y., Long, Z., & He, Y. (2021). Effect of Protein-Rich Breakfast on Subsequent Energy Intake and Subjective Appetite in Children and Adolescents: Systematic Review and Meta-Analysis of Randomized Controlled Trials. *Nutrients*, 13(8), 2840. https://doi.org/10.3390/nu13082840

106. Dhillon, J., Craig, B. A., Leidy, H. J., Amankwaah, A. F., Osei-Boadi Anguah, K., Jacobs, A., Jones, B. L., Jones, J. B., Keeler, C. L., Keller, C. E., McCrory, M. A., Rivera, R. L., Slebodnik, M., Mattes, R. D., & Tucker, R. M. (2016). The Effects of Increased Protein Intake on Fullness: A Meta-Analysis and Its Limitations. *Journal of the Academy of Nutrition and Dietetics*, 116(6), 968–83. https://doi.org/10.1016/j.jand.2016.01.003

107. Khaing, I. K., Tahara, Y., Chimed-Ochir, O., Shibata, S., & Kubo, T. (2024). Effect of Breakfast Protein Intake on Muscle Mass and Strength in Adults: A Scoping Review. *Nutrition Reviews*, nuad167. https://doi.org/10.1093/nutrit/nuad167

108. Gortmaker, S. L., Must, A., Sobol, A. M., Peterson, K., Colditz, G. A., & Dietz, W. H. (1996). Television Viewing as a Cause of Increasing Obesity Among Children in the United States, 1986–1990. *Archives of Pediatrics & Adolescent Medicine*, 150(4), 356–62. https://doi.org/10.1001/archpedi.1996.02170290022003

109. Russell, S. J., et al. The Effect of Screen Advertising on Children's Dietary Intake: A Systematic Review and Meta-Analysis.

110. Sadeghirad, B., Duhaney, T., Motaghipisheh, S., Campbell, N. R., & Johnston, B. C. (2016). Influence of Unhealthy Food and Beverage Marketing on Children's Dietary Intake and Preference: A Systematic Review and Meta-Analysis of Randomized Trials.

Obesity Reviews : An Official Journal of the International Association for the Study of Obesity, 17(10), 945–959. https://doi.org/10.1111/obr.12445

111. Blass, E. M., Anderson, D. R., Kirkorian, H. L., Pempek, T. A., Price, I., & Koleini, M. F. (2006). On the Road to Obesity: Television Viewing Increases Intake of High-Density Foods. *Physiology & Behavior*, 88(4-5), 597–604. https://doi.org/10.1016/j.physbeh.2006.05.035

112. Ibid.

113. Ding, L., Hamid, N., Shepherd, D., & Kantono, K. (2019). How Is Satiety Affected When Consuming Food While Working on a Computer? *Nutrients*, 11(7), 1545. https://doi.org/10.3390/nu11071545

114. La Marra, M., Caviglia, G., & Perrella, R. (2020). Using Smartphones When Eating Increases Caloric Intake in Young People: An Overview of the Literature. *Frontiers in Psychology*, 11, 587886. https://doi.org/10.3389/fpsyg.2020.587886

115. Robinson, E., Aveyard, P., Daley, A., Jolly, K., Lewis, A., Lycett, D., & Higgs, S. (2013). Eating Attentively: A Systematic Review and Meta-Analysis of the Effect of Food Intake Memory and Awareness on Eating. *The American Journal of Clinical Nutrition*, 97(4), 728–42. https://doi.org/10.3945/ajcn.112.045245

116. Ohkuma, T., Hirakawa, Y., Nakamura, U., Kiyohara, Y., Kitazono, T., & Ninomiya, T. (2015). Association Between Eating Rate and Obesity: A Systematic Review and Meta-Analysis. *International Journal of Obesity*, 39(11), 1589–96. https://doi.org/10.1038/ijo.2015.96

117. Yuan, S. Q., Liu, Y. M., Liang, W., Li, F. F., Zeng, Y., Liu, Y. Y., Huang, S. Z., He, Q. Y., Quach, B., Jiao, J., Baker, J. S., & Yang, Y. D. (2021). Association Between Eating Speed and Metabolic Syndrome: A Systematic Review and Meta-Analysis. *Frontiers in Nutrition*, 8, 700936. https://doi.org/10.3389/fnut.2021.700936

118. Robinson, E., Almiron-Roig, E., Rutters, F., De Graaf, C., Forde, C. G., Tudur Smith, C., Nolan, S. J., & Jebb, S. A. (2014). A Systematic Review and Meta-Analysis Examining the Effect of Eating Rate on Energy Intake and Hunger. *The American Journal of Clinical Nutrition*, 100(1), 123–51. https://doi.org/10.3945/ajcn.113.081745

119. Hunter, J. A., Hollands, G. J., Couturier, D. L., & Marteau, T. M. (2018). Effect of Snack-Food Proximity on Intake in General Population Samples With Higher and Lower Cognitive Resource. *Appetite*, 121, 337–47. https://doi.org/10.1016/j.appet.2017.11.101

120. Vogel, C., Crozier, S., Penn-Newman, D., Ball, K., Moon, G., Lord, J., Cooper, C., & Baird, J.

(2021). Altering Product Placement to Create a Healthier Layout in Supermarkets: Outcomes on Store Sales, Customer Purchasing, and Diet in a Prospective Matched Controlled Cluster Study. *PloS Medicine*, 18(9), e1003729. https://doi.org/10.1371/journal. pmed.1003729

121. Thorndike, A. N., et al. A 2-Phase Labeling and Choice Architecture Intervention to Improve Healthy Food and Beverage Choices.

122. Adjoian, T., Dannefer, R., Willingham, C., Brathwaite, C., & Franklin, S. (2017). Healthy Checkout Lines: A Study in Urban Supermarkets. *Journal of Nutrition Education and Behavior*, 49(8), 615–22.e1. https://doi.org/10.1016/j. jneb.2017.02.004

123. Nakamura, R., Pechey, R., Suhrcke, M., Jebb, S. A., & Marteau, T. M. (2014). Sales Impact of Displaying Alcoholic and Non-alcoholic Beverages in End-of-Aisle Locations: An Observational Study. *Social Science & Medicine*, 108(100), 68–73. https://doi.org/10.1016/j. socscimed.2014.02.032

124. Arno, A., & Thomas, S. (2016). The Efficacy of Nudge Theory Strategies in Influencing Adult Dietary Behaviour: A Systematic Review and Meta-Analysis. *BMC Public Health*, 16, 676. https://doi. org/10.1186/s12889-016-3272-x

125. Neve, K. L., & Isaacs, A. (2022). How Does the Food Environment Influence People Engaged in Weight Management? A Systematic Review and Thematic Synthesis of the Qualitative Literature. *Obesity Reviews: An Official Journal of the International Association for the Study of Obesity*, 23(3), e13398. https://doi. org/10.1111/obr.13398

126. Blazey, P., Habibi, A., Hassen, N., Friedman, D., Khan, K. M., & Ardern, C. L. (2023). The Effects of Eating Frequency on Changes in Body Composition and Cardiometabolic Health in Adults: A Systematic Review With Meta-Analysis of Randomized Trials. *The International Journal of Behavioral Nutrition and Physical Activity*, 20(1), 133. https://doi.org/10.1186/ s12966-023-01532-z

127. Westenhoefer, J., von Falck, B., Stellfeldt, A., & Fintelmann, S. (2004). Behavioural Correlates of Successful Weight Reduction Over 3 Y. Results From the Lean Habits Study. *International Journal of Obesity and Related Metabolic Disorders: Journal of the International Association for the Study of Obesity*, 28(2), 334–5. https://doi.org/10.1038/ sj.ijo.0802530

128. Zendegui, E. A., West, J. A., & Zandberg, L. J. (2014). Binge Eating Frequency and Regular Eating Adherence: The Role of Eating Pattern in Cognitive Behavioral Guided Self-Help. *Eating*

*Behaviors*, 15(2), 241–3. https://doi.org/10.1016/j.eatbeh.2014.03.002

129. Gorin, A. A., Phelan, S., Wing, R. R., & Hill, J. O. (2004). Promoting Long-Term Weight Control: Does Dieting Consistency Matter? *International Journal of Obesity and Related Metabolic Disorders: Journal of the International Association for the Study of Obesity*, 28(2), 278–81. https://doi.org/10.1038/sj.ijo.0802550

130. Jorge, R., Santos, I., Teixeira, V. H., & Teixeira, P. J. (2019). Does Diet Strictness Level During Weekends and Holiday Periods Influence 1-Year Follow-Up Weight Loss Maintenance? Evidence From the Portuguese Weight Control Registry. *Nutrition Journal*, 18(1), 3. https://doi.org/10.1186/s12937-019-0430-x

131. Ibid.

## Chapter 6

1. Feil, K., Fritsch, J., & Rhodes, R. E. (2023). The Intention-Behaviour Gap in Physical Activity: A Systematic Review and Meta-Analysis of the Action Control Framework. *British Journal of Sports Medicine*, 57(19), 1265–71. https://doi.org/10.1136/bjsports-2022-106640

2. MacLean, P. S., Wing, R. R., Davidson, T., Epstein, L., Goodpaster, B., Hall, K. D., Levin, B. E., Perri, M. G., Rolls, B. J., Rosenbaum, M., Rothman, A. J., & Ryan, D. (2015). NIH Working Group Report: Innovative Research to Improve Maintenance of Weight Loss. *Obesity*, 23(1), 7–15. https://doi.org/10.1002/oby.20967

3. Pigsborg, K., Kalea, A. Z., De Dominicis, S., & Magkos, F. (2023). Behavioral and Psychological Factors Affecting Weight Loss Success. *Current Obesity Reports*, 12(3), 223–30. https://doi.org/10.1007/s13679-023-00511-6

4. Bidgood, J., & Buckroyd, J. (2005). An Exploration of Obese Adults' Experience of Attempting to Lose Weight and to Maintain a Reduced Weight. *Counselling and Psychotherapy Research*, 5(3), 221–9. https://doi.org/10.1080/17441690500310395

5. Byrne, S., Cooper, Z., & Fairburn, C. (2003). Weight Maintenance and Relapse in Obesity: A Qualitative Study. *International Journal of Obesity and Related Metabolic Disorders: Journal of the International Association for the Study of Obesity*, 27(8), 955–62. https://doi.org/10.1038/sj.ijo.0802305

6. Ohsiek, S., & Williams, M. (2011). Psychological Factors Influencing Weight Loss Maintenance: *An Integrative Literature Review*. *Journal of the American Academy of Nurse Practitioners*, 23(11), 592–601. https://doi.org/10.1111/j.1745-7599.2011.00647.x

7. Gormally, J., Rardin, D., & Black, S. (1980). Correlates of Successful Response to a Behavioral

Weight Control Clinic. *Journal of Counseling Psychology*, 27(2), 179–91. https://doi.org/10.1037/0022-0167.27.2.179

8. Dakanalis, A., et al. The Association of Emotional Eating With Overweight/Obesity, Depression, Anxiety/Stress, and Dietary Patterns: A Review of the Current Clinical Evidence.

9. Fuente González, C. E., et al. Relationship Between Emotional Eating, Consumption of Hyperpalatable Energy-Dense Foods, and Indicators of Nutritional Status: A Systematic Review.

10. Micanti, F., Iasevoli, F., Cucciniello, C., Costabile, R., Loiarro, G., Pecoraro, G., Pasanisi, F., Rossetti, G., & Galletta, D. (2017). The Relationship Between Emotional Regulation and Eating Behaviour: A Multidimensional Analysis of Obesity Psychopathology. *Eating and Weight Disorders—Studies on Anorexia, Bulimia, and Obesity*, 22(1), 105–15. https://doi.org/10.1007/s40519-016-0275-7

11. Frayn, M., Livshits, S., & Knäuper, B. (2018). Emotional Eating and Weight Regulation: A Qualitative Study of Compensatory Behaviors and Concerns. *Journal of Eating Disorders*, 6, 23. https://doi.org/10.1186/s40337-018-0210-6

12. Ingels, J. S., & Zizzi, S. (2018). A Qualitative Analysis of the Role of Emotions in Different Patterns of Long-Term Weight Loss. *Psychology & Health*, 33(8), 1014–27. https://doi.org/10.1080/08870446.2018.1453511

13. Czepczor-Bernat, K., & Brytek-Matera, A. (2021). The Impact of Food-Related Behaviours and Emotional Functioning on Body Mass Index in an Adult Sample. *Eating and Weight Disorders—Studies on Anorexia, Bulimia, and Obesity*, 26(1), 323–9. https://doi.org/10.1007/s40519-020-00853-3

14. Ibid.

15. Smith, J., Ang, X. Q., Giles, E. L., & Traviss-Turner, G. (2023). Emotional Eating Interventions for Adults Living With Overweight or Obesity: A Systematic Review and Meta-Analysis. *International Journal of Environmental Research and Public Health*, 20(3), 2722. https://doi.org/10.3390/ijerph20032722

16. Weinbach, N., Barzilay, G., & Cohen, N. (2022). Cognitive Reappraisal Reduces the Influence of Threat on Food Craving. *Affective Science*, 3(4), 818–26. https://doi.org/10.1007/s42761-022-00141-6

17. Gerosa, M., Canessa, N., Morawetz, C., & Mattavelli, G. (2024). Cognitive Reappraisal of Food Craving and Emotions: A Coordinate-Based Meta-Analysis of fMRI Studies. *Social Cognitive and Affective Neuroscience*, 19(1), nsado77. https://doi.org/10.1093/scan/nsado77

18. Fernandes, J., Ferreira-Santos, F., Miller, K., & Torres, S. (2018). Emotional Processing in Obesity: A Systematic Review and Exploratory Meta-Analysis. *Obesity Reviews: An Official Journal of the International Association for the Study of Obesity*, 19(1), 111–20. https://doi.org/10.1111/obr.12607

19. Favieri, F., Marini, A., & Casagrande, M. (2021). Emotional Regulation and Overeating Behaviors in Children and Adolescents: A Systematic Review. *Behavioral Sciences*, 11(1), 11. https://doi.org/10.3390/bs11010011

20. Ranney, R. M., Bruehlman-Senecal, E., & Ayduk, O. (2017). Comparing the Effects of Three Online Cognitive Reappraisal Trainings on Well-Being. *Journal of Happiness Studies*, 18, 1319–38. https://doi.org/10.1007/s10902-016-9779-0

21. Herman, C. P., & Mack, D. (1975). Restrained and Unrestrained Eating. *Journal of Personality*, 43(4), 647–60. https://doi.org/10.1111/j.1467-6494.1975.tb00727.x

22. Polivy, J., & Herman, C. P. (2020). Overeating in Restrained and Unrestrained Eaters. *Frontiers in Nutrition*, 7, 30. https://doi.org/10.3389/fnut.2020.00030

23. Oshio, A. (2009). Development and Validation of the Dichotomous Thinking Inventory. *Social Behavior and Personality: An International Journal*, 37(6), 729–42. https://doi.org/10.2224/sbp.2009.37.6.729

24. Ohsiek, S., & Williams, M. Psychological Factors Influencing Weight Loss Maintenance.

25. Byrne, S. M., Cooper, Z., & Fairburn, C. G. (2004). Psychological Predictors of Weight Regain in Obesity. *Behaviour Research and Therapy*, 42(11), 1341–56. https://doi.org/10.1016/j.brat.2003.09.004

26. Palascha, A., Van Kleef, E., & Van Trijp, H. C. (2015). How Does Thinking in Black and White Terms Relate to Eating Behavior and Weight Regain? *Journal of Health Psychology*, 20(5), 638–48. https://doi.org/10.1177/1359105315573440

27. Marshall, C., Reay, R., & Bowman, A. R. (2024). Weight Loss After Weight-Loss Surgery: The Mediating Role of Dichotomous Thinking. *Obesity Surgery*, 34(5), 1523–7. https://doi.org/10.1007/s11695-024-07122-7

28. Byrne, S. M., Allen, K. L., Dove, E. R., Watt, F. J., & Nathan, P. R. (2008). The Reliability and Validity of the Dichotomous Thinking in Eating Disorders Scale. *Eating Behaviors*, 9(2), 154–62. https://doi.org/10.1016/j.eatbeh.2007.07.002

29. He, X. (2016). When Perfectionism Leads to Imperfect Consumer Choices: The Role of Dichotomous Thinking. *Journal of Consumer*

*Psychology*, 26(1), 98–104. https://doi.org/10.1016/j.jcps.2015.04.002

30. Goldstein, S. P., Evans, E. W., Espel-Huynh, H. M., Goldstein, C. M., Karchere-Sun, R., & Thomas, J. G. (2022). Dietary Lapses Are Associated With Meaningful Elevations in Daily Caloric Intake and Added Sugar Consumption During a Lifestyle Modification Intervention. *Obesity Science & Practice*, 8(4), 442–54. https://doi.org/10.1002/osp4.587

31. Carels, R. A., Hoffman, J., Collins, A., Raber, A. C., Cacciapaglia, H., & O'Brien, W. H. (2001). Ecological Momentary Assessment of Temptation and Lapse in Dieting. *Eating Behaviors*, 2(4), 307–21. https://doi.org/10.1016/s1471-0153(01)00037-X

32. Carels, R. A., Douglass, O. M., Cacciapaglia, H. M., & O'Brien, W. H. (2004). An Ecological Momentary Assessment of Relapse Crises in Dieting. *Journal of Consulting and Clinical Psychology*, 72(2), 341–8. https://doi.org/10.1037/0022–006X.72.2.341

33. Neff, K. D. (2023). Self-Compassion: Theory, Method, Research, and Intervention. *Annual Review of Psychology*, 74, 193–218. https://doi.org/10.1146/annurev-psych-032420-031047

34. Hagerman, C. J., Ehmann, M. M., Taylor, L. C., & Forman, E. M. (2023). The Role of Self-Compassion and Its Individual Components in Adaptive Responses to Dietary Lapses. *Appetite*, 190, 107009. https://doi.org/10.1016/j.appet.2023.107009

35. Adams, C. E., & Leary, M. R. (2007). Promoting Self-Compassionate Attitudes Toward Eating Among Restrictive and Guilty Eaters. *Journal of Social and Clinical Psychology*, 26(10), 1120–44. https://doi.org/10.1521/jscp.2007.26.10.1120

36. Rahimi-Ardabili, H., Reynolds, R., Vartanian, L. R., McLeod, L. V. D., & Zwar, N. (2018). A Systematic Review of the Efficacy of Interventions That Aim to Increase Self-Compassion on Nutrition Habits, Eating Behaviours, Body Weight and Body Image. *Mindfulness*, 9, 388–400. https://doi.org/10.1007/s12671-017-0804-0

37. Brenton-Peters, J., Consedine, N. S., Boggiss, A., Wallace-Boyd, K., Roy, R., & Serlachius, A. (2021). Self-Compassion in Weight Management: A Systematic Review. *Journal of Psychosomatic Research*, 150, 110617. https://doi.org/10.1016/j.jpsychores.2021.110617

38. Byrne, S., et al. Weight Maintenance and Relapse in Obesity.

39. Teixeira, P. J., Carraça, E. V., Marques, M. M., Rutter, H., Oppert, J. M., De Bourdeaudhuij, I., Lakerveld, J., & Brug, J. (2015). Successful Behavior Change

in Obesity Interventions in Adults: A Systematic Review of Self-Regulation Mediators. *BMC Medicine*, 13, 84. https://doi.org/10.1186/s12916-015-0323-6

40. Rafiei, N., & Gill, T. (2018). Identification of Factors Contributing to Successful Self-Directed Weight Loss: A Qualitative Study. *Journal of Human Nutrition and Dietetics: The Official Journal of the British Dietetic Association*, 31(3), 329–36. https://doi.org/10.1111/jhn.12522

41. Byrne, S., et al. Weight Maintenance and Relapse in Obesity.

42. Ohsiek, S., & Williams, M. Psychological Factors Influencing Weight Loss Maintenance.

43. Frayn, M., et al. Emotional Eating and Weight Regulation.

44. Teixeira, P. J., et al. Successful Behavior Change in Obesity Interventions in Adults.

45. Dalle Grave, R., Centis, E., Marzocchi, R., El Ghoch, M., & Marchesini, G. (2013). Major Factors for Facilitating Change in Behavioral Strategies to Reduce Obesity. *Psychology Research and Behavior Management*, 6, 101–10. https://doi.org/10.2147/PRBM.S40460

46. Shriver, L. H., Dollar, J. M., Calkins, S. D., Keane, S. P., Shanahan, L., & Wideman, L. (2020). Emotional Eating in Adolescence: Effects of Emotion Regulation, Weight Status and Negative Body Image. *Nutrients*, 13(1), 79. https://doi.org/10.3390/nu13010079

## Chapter 7

1. Wadden, T. A., & Foster, G. D. (2000). Behavioral Treatment of Obesity. *The Medical Clinics of North America*, 84(2), 441–61. https://doi.org/10.1016/s0025-7125(05)70230-3

2. Bravata, D. M., Smith-Spangler, C., Sundaram, V., Gienger, A. L., Lin, N., Lewis, R., Stave, C. D., Olkin, I., & Sirard, J. R. (2007). Using Pedometers to Increase Physical Activity and Improve Health: A Systematic Review. *JAMA*, 298(19), 2296–304. https://doi.org/10.1001/jama.298.19.2296

3. Longhini, J., Marzaro, C., Bargeri, S., Palese, A., Dell'Isola, A., Turolla, A., Pillastrini, P., Battista, S., Castellini, G., Cook, C., Gianola, S., & Rossettini, G. (2024). Wearable Devices to Improve Physical Activity and Reduce Sedentary Behaviour: An Umbrella Review. *Sports Medicine—Open*, 10(1), 9. https://doi.org/10.1186/s40798-024-00678-9

4. Rosenbaum, M., Hirsch, J., Gallagher, D. A., & Leibel, R. L. (2008). Long-Term Persistence of Adaptive Thermogenesis in Subjects Who Have Maintained a Reduced Body Weight. *The American Journal of Clinical*

*Nutrition*, 88(4), 906–12. https://doi.org/10.1093/ajcn/88.4.906

5. Ostendorf, D. M., Caldwell, A. E., Creasy, S. A., Pan, Z., Lyden, K., Bergouignan, A., MacLean, P. S., Wyatt, H. R., Hill, J. O., Melanson, E. L., & Catenacci, V. A. (2019). Physical Activity Energy Expenditure and Total Daily Energy Expenditure in Successful Weight Loss Maintainers. *Obesity*, 27(3), 496–504. https://doi.org/10.1002/oby.22373

6. Ibid.

7. Sperduto, W. A., Thompson, H. S., & O'Brien, R. M. (1986). The Effect of Target Behavior Monitoring on Weight Loss and Completion Rate in a Behavior Modification Program for Weight Reduction. *Addictive Behaviors*, 11(3), 337–40. https://doi.org/10.1016/0306-4603(86)90060-2

8. Baker, R. C., & Kirschenbaum, D. S. (1993). Self-Monitoring May Be Necessary for Successful Weight Control. *Behavior Therapy*, 24(3), 377–94. https://doi.org/10.1016/S0005-7894(05)80212–6

9. Carter, M. C., Burley, V. J., Nykjaer, C., & Cade, J. E. (2013). Adherence to a Smartphone Application for Weight Loss Compared to Website and Paper Diary: Pilot Randomized Controlled Trial. *Journal of Medical Internet Research*, 15(4), e32. https://doi.org/10.2196/jmir.2283

10. Ferrara, G., Kim, J., Lin, S., Hua, J., & Seto, E. (2019). A Focused Review of Smartphone Diet-Tracking Apps: Usability, Functionality, Coherence With Behavior Change Theory, and Comparative Validity of Nutrient Intake and Energy Estimates. *JMIR mHealth and uHealth*, 7(5), e9232. https://doi.org/10.2196/mhealth.9232

11. Rumbo-Rodríguez, L., Sánchez-SanSegundo, M., Ruiz-Robledillo, N., Albaladejo-Blázquez, N., Ferrer-Cascales, R., & Zaragoza-Martí, A. (2020). Use of Technology-Based Interventions in the Treatment of Patients With Overweight and Obesity: A Systematic Review. *Nutrients*, 12(12), 3634. https://doi.org/10.3390/nu12123634

12. Semper, H. M., Povey, R., & Clark-Carter, D. (2016). A Systematic Review of the Effectiveness of Smartphone Applications That Encourage Dietary Self-Regulatory Strategies for Weight Loss in Overweight and Obese Adults. *Obesity Reviews: An Official Journal of the International Association for the Study of Obesity*, 17(9), 895–906. https://doi.org/10.1111/obr.12428

13. Kupila, S. K. E., Joki, A., Suojanen, L. U., & Pietiläinen, K. H. (2023). The Effectiveness of eHealth Interventions for Weight Loss and Weight Loss Maintenance in Adults With Overweight or Obesity: A Systematic Review of Systematic Reviews. *Current Obesity Reports*, 12(3),

371–94. https://doi.org/10.1007/s13679-023-00515-2

14. US Food & Drug Administration (2018). Guidance for Industry: Guide for Developing and Using Data Bases for Nutrition Labeling. Retrieved from https://www.fda.gov/regulatory-information/search-fda-guidance-documents/guidance-industry-guide-developing-and-using-data-bases-nutrition-labeling#N_1_

15. Urban, L. E., Dallal, G. E., Robinson, L. M., Ausman, L. M., Saltzman, E., & Roberts, S. B. (2010). The Accuracy of Stated Energy Contents of Reduced-Energy, Commercially Prepared Foods. *Journal of the American Dietetic Association*, 110(1), 116–23. https://doi.org/10.1016/j.jada.2009.10.003

16. Levinson, C. A., Fewell, L., & Brosof, L. C. (2017). My Fitness Pal Calorie Tracker Usage in the Eating Disorders. *Eating Behaviors*, 27, 14–16. https://doi.org/10.1016/j.eatbeh.2017.08.003

17. Simpson, C. C., & Mazzeo, S. E. (2017). Calorie Counting and Fitness Tracking Technology: Associations With Eating Disorder Symptomatology. *Eating Behaviors*, 26, 89–92. https://doi.org/10.1016/j.eatbeh.2017.02.002

18. Linardon, J., & Messer, M. (2019). My Fitness Pal Usage in Men: Associations With Eating Disorder Symptoms and Psychosocial Impairment. *Eating Behaviors*,

33, 13–17. https://doi.org/10.1016/j.eatbeh.2019.02.003

19. Romano, K. A., Swanbrow Becker, M. A., Colgary, C. D., & Magnuson, A. (2018). Helpful or Harmful? The Comparative Value of Self-Weighing and Calorie Counting Versus Intuitive Eating on the Eating Disorder Symptomology of College Students. *Eating and Weight Disorders—Studies on Anorexia, Bulimia, and Obesity*, 23(6), 841–8. https://doi.org/10.1007/s40519-018-0562-6

20. Jospe, M. R., Brown, R. C., Williams, S. M., Roy, M., Meredith-Jones, K. A., & Taylor, R. W. (2018). Self-Monitoring Has No Adverse Effect on Disordered Eating in Adults Seeking Treatment for Obesity. *Obesity Science & Practice*, 4(3), 283–8. https://doi.org/10.1002/osp4.168

21. Hahn, S. L., Kaciroti, N., Eisenberg, D., Weeks, H. M., Bauer, K. W., & Sonneville, K. R. (2021). Introducing Dietary Self-Monitoring to Undergraduate Women via a Calorie Counting App Has No Effect on Mental Health or Health Behaviors: Results From a Randomized Controlled Trial. *Journal of the Academy of Nutrition and Dietetics*, 121(12), 2377–88. https://doi.org/10.1016/j.jand.2021.06.311

22. Semper, H. M. et al. A Systematic Review of the Effectiveness of Smartphone Applications That Encourage Dietary Self-Regulatory

Strategies for Weight Loss in Overweight and Obese Adults.

23. Kupila, S. K. E. et al. The Effectiveness of eHealth Interventions for Weight Loss and Weight Loss Maintenance in Adults With Overweight or Obesity.

24. Burke, L. E., Wang, J., & Sevick, M. A. (2011). Self-Monitoring in Weight Loss: A Systematic Review of the Literature. *Journal of the American Dietetic Association*, 111(1), 92–102. https://doi.org/10.1016/j.jada.2010.10.008

25. Raber, M., Liao, Y., Rara, A., Schembre, S. M., Krause, K. J., Strong, L., Daniel-MacDougall, C., & Basen-Engquist, K. (2021). A Systematic Review of the Use of Dietary Self-Monitoring in Behavioural Weight Loss Interventions: Delivery, Intensity and Effectiveness. *Public Health Nutrition*, 24(17), 5885–913. https://doi.org/10.1017/S136898002100358X

26. Berry, R., Kassavou, A., & Sutton, S. (2021). Does Self-Monitoring Diet and Physical Activity Behaviors Using Digital Technology Support Adults With Obesity or Overweight to Lose Weight? A Systematic Literature Review With Meta-Analysis. *Obesity Reviews: An Official Journal of the International Association for the Study of Obesity*, 22(10), e13306. https://doi.org/10.1111/obr.13306

27. Krukowski, R. A., Harvey, J., Borden, J., Stansbury, M. L., & West, D. S. (2022). Expert Opinions on Reducing Dietary Self-Monitoring Burden and Maintaining Efficacy in Weight Loss Programs: A Delphi Study. *Obesity Science & Practice*, 8(4), 401–10. https://doi.org/10.1002/osp4.586

28. Helsel, D. L., Jakicic, J. M., & Otto, A. D. (2007). Comparison of Techniques for Self-Monitoring Eating and Exercise Behaviors on Weight Loss in a Correspondence-Based Intervention. *Journal of the American Dietetic Association*, 107(10), 1807–10. https://doi.org/10.1016/j.jada.2007.07.014

29. Crane, M. M., Lutes, L. D., Ward, D. S., Bowling, J. M., & Tate, D. F. (2015). A Randomized Trial Testing the Efficacy of a Novel Approach to Weight Loss Among Men With Overweight and Obesity. *Obesity*, 23(12), 2398–405. https://doi.org/10.1002/oby.21265

30. Tate, D. F., Quesnel, D. A., Lutes, L., Hatley, K. E., Nezami, B. T., Wojtanowski, A. C., Pinto, A. M., Power, J., Diamond, M., Polzien, K., & Foster, G. (2020). Examination of a Partial Dietary Self-Monitoring Approach for Behavioral Weight Management. *Obesity Science & Practice*, 6(4), 353–64. https://doi.org/10.1002/osp4.416

31. Nezami, B. T., Hurley, L., Power, J., Valle, C. G., & Tate, D. F. (2022).

A Pilot Randomized Trial of Simplified Versus Standard Calorie Dietary Self-Monitoring in a Mobile Weight Loss Intervention. *Obesity*, 30(3), 628–38. https://doi.org/10.1002/oby.23377

32. Patel, M. L., Cleare, A. E., Smith, C. M., Rosas, L. G., & King, A. C. (2022). Detailed Versus Simplified Dietary Self-Monitoring in a Digital Weight Loss Intervention Among Racial and Ethnic Minority Adults: Fully Remote, Randomized Pilot Study. *JMIR Formative Research*, 6(12), e42191. https://doi.org/10.2196/42191

33. Adapted from Beeken, R. J., Leurent, B., Vickerstaff, V., Wilson, R., Croker, H., Morris, S., Omar, R. Z., Nazareth, I., & Wardle, J. (2017). A Brief Intervention for Weight Control Based on Habit-Formation Theory Delivered Through Primary Care: Results From a Randomised Controlled Trial. *International Journal of Obesity*, 41(2), 246–54. https://doi.org/10.1038/ijo.2016.206

34. Burke, L. E., et al. Self-Monitoring in Weight Loss.

35. Ibid.

36. VanWormer, J. J., French, S. A., Pereira, M. A., & Welsh, E. M. (2008). The Impact of Regular Self-Weighing on Weight Management: A Systematic Literature Review. *The International Journal of Behavioral Nutrition and Physical Activity*, 5, 54. https://doi.org/10.1186/1479-5868-5-54

37. Zheng, Y., Klem, M. L., Sereika, S. M., Danford, C. A., Ewing, L. J., & Burke, L. E. (2015). Self-Weighing in Weight Management: A Systematic Literature Review. *Obesity*, 23(2), 256–65. https://doi.org/10.1002/oby.20946

38. Shieh, C., Knisely, M. R., Clark, D., & Carpenter, J. S. (2016). Self-Weighing in Weight Management Interventions: A Systematic Review of Literature. *Obesity Research & Clinical Practice*, 10(5), 493–519. https://doi.org/10.1016/j.orcp.2016.01.004

39. Paixão, C., Dias, C. M., Jorge, R., Carraça, E. V., Yannakoulia, M., De Zwaan, M., Soini, S., Hill, J. O., Teixeira, P. J., & Santos, I. (2020). Successful Weight Loss Maintenance: A Systematic Review of Weight Control Registries. *Obesity Reviews: An Official Journal of the International Association for the Study of Obesity*, 21(5), e13003. https://doi.org/10.1111/obr.13003

40. Hahn, S. L., Pacanowski, C. R., Loth, K. A., Miller, J., Eisenberg, M. E., & Neumark-Sztainer, D. (2021). Self-Weighing Among Young Adults: Who Weighs Themselves and for Whom Does Weighing Affect Mood? A Cross-Sectional Study of a Population-Based Sample. *Journal of Eating Disorders*, 9(1), 37. https://doi.org/10.1186/s40337-021-00391-y

41. Mintz, L. B., Awad, G. H., Stinson, R. D., Bledman, R. A., Coker, A. D., Kashubeck-West, S., & Connelly, K. (2013). Weighing and Body Monitoring Among College Women: The Scale Number as an Emotional Barometer. *Journal of College Student Psychotherapy*, 27(1), 78–91. https://doi.org/10.108 0/87568225.2013.739039

42. Ogden, J., & Whyman, C. (1997). The Effect of Repeated Weighing on Psychological State. *European Eating Disorders Review: The Professional Journal of the Eating Disorders Association*, 5(2), 121–30. https://doi.org/10.1002/(SICI) 1099-0968(199706)5:2<121::AID- ERV167>3.0.CO;2-N

43. Hagerman, C. J., Onu, M. C., Crane, N. T., Butryn, M. L., & Forman, E. M. (2024). Psychological and Behavioral Responses to Daily Weight Gain During Behavioral Weight Loss Treatment. *Journal of Behavioral Medicine*, 47(3), 492–503. https://doi.org/10.1007/ s10865-024-00476-4

44. Tylka, T. L., Annunziato, R. A., Burgard, D., Daníelsdóttir, S., Shuman, E., Davis, C., & Calogero, R. M. (2014). The Weight-Inclusive Versus Weight-Normative Approach to Health: Evaluating the Evidence for Prioritizing Well- Being Over Weight Loss. *Journal of Obesity*, 983495. https://doi. org/10.1155/2014/983495

45. Dugmore, J. A., Winten, C. G., Niven, H. E., & Bauer, J. (2020). Effects of Weight-Neutral Approaches Compared With Traditional Weight-Loss Approaches on Behavioral, Physical, and Psychological Health Outcomes: A Systematic Review and Meta-Analysis. *Nutrition Reviews*, 78(1), 39–55. https://doi. org/10.1093/nutrit/nuz020

46. Gaesser, G. A., & Angadi, S. S. (2021). Obesity Treatment: Weight Loss Versus Increasing Fitness and Physical Activity for Reducing Health Risks. *iScience*, 24(10), 102995. https://doi.org/10.1016/j. isci.2021.102995

47. Jospe, M. R. et al. Self-Monitoring Has No Adverse Effect on Disordered Eating in Adults Seeking Treatment for Obesity.

48. Fahey, M. C., Klesges, R. C., Kocak, M., Wayne Talcott, G., & Krukowski, R. A. (2018). Changes in the Perceptions of Self-Weighing Across Time in a Behavioral Weight Loss Intervention. *Obesity*, 26(10), 1566–75. https://doi.org/10.1002/ oby.22275

49. Pacanowski, C. R., Linde, J. A., & Neumark-Sztainer, D. (2015). Self-Weighing: Helpful or Harmful for Psychological Well-Being? A Review of the Literature. *Current Obesity Reports*, 4(1), 65–72. https:// doi.org/10.1007/s13679-015-0142-2

50. Benn, Y., Webb, T. L., Chang, B. P., & Harkin, B. (2016). What Is the

Psychological Impact of Self-Weighing? A Meta-Analysis. *Health Psychology Review*, 10(2), 187–203. https://doi.org/10.1080/17437199.2016.1138871

51. Kiernan, M., Brown, S. D., Schoffman, D. E., Lee, K., King, A. C., Taylor, C. B., Schleicher, N. C., & Perri, M. G. (2013). Promoting Healthy Weight With "Stability Skills First": A Randomized Trial. *Journal of Consulting and Clinical Psychology*, 81(2), 336–46. https://doi.org/10.1037/a0030544

52. Ross, R., Neeland, I. J., Yamashita, S., Shai, I., Seidell, J., Magni, P., Santos, R. D., Arsenault, B., Cuevas, A., Hu, F. B., Griffin, B. A., Zambon, A., Barter, P., Fruchart, J. C., Eckel, R. H., Matsuzawa, Y., & Després, J. P. (2020). Waist Circumference as a Vital Sign in Clinical Practice: A Consensus Statement From the IAS and ICCR Working Group on Visceral Obesity. *Nature Reviews: Endocrinology*, 16(3), 177–89. https://doi.org/10.1038/s41574-019-0310-7

53. Jayedi, A., Soltani, S., Zargar, M. S., Khan, T. A., & Shab-Bidar, S. (2020). Central Fatness and Risk of All Cause Mortality: Systematic Review and Dose-Response Meta-Analysis of 72 Prospective Cohort Studies. *BMJ*, 370:m3324. https://doi.org/10.1136/bmj.m3324

# Index

# Acknowledgments

Thank you for taking the time to read this book. It is impossible for me to adequately express how grateful I am to everyone involved, but here is my best shot.

As someone who has always been incredibly shy and lacking in self-belief, the fortunate position I now find myself in simply wouldn't have been possible without your amazing support.

I didn't ever think I would write a book, let alone two. Not because I didn't want to, but simply because I didn't think I had the talent to be successful. Would any of you care if I wrote a book? Would any of you want to spend hours of your precious time reading what I had to say? I severely doubted it.

My wife was the first person to help turn this around. When we first met, she seemed bewildered that I questioned my ability. She had already known of me as someone who had been putting free content on social media for over a decade, and she assured me that this was testament to how many of you were interested in what I had to say. She became my biggest inspiration and loudest cheerleader all at once. Without her, I would never have started writing at all. Having someone wholeheartedly believe in you more than you have ever believed in yourself can be powerful enough to turn your whole life around.

The goal for my first book, *Everything Fat Loss*, was simple: to take the most popular topic in the fitness industry (losing body fat) and write the best fucking book and scientific resource I could. If it did really well, I could hopefully help disrupt an industry that has more than its fair share of dangerous misinformation and shady characters who are happy to lie to you to try and get their hands on your hard-earned money.

Once I had written my first draft, a whopping 140,000 words (which any author will tell you is more like two books rather than one), a good friend of mine, Luke Betts, affectionately told me that I was being a dickhead for spending nearly three years writing a book to only make it available online as a digital PDF. In his words, "You should gamble on yourself. Do it properly, pay to get it printed as a self-published book and let people physically hold the thing you have put so much blood, sweat and tears into." Without his confidence, my first book would never have been printed, would have never become an online best-seller, and I would never have caught the attention of several of the world's biggest publishers.

When Helena, a commissioning editor at Octopus Books, emailed me, it was clear that not only had she read my first book in full, something that no other publisher had done, but she loved it and understood my intense passion for this topic. When she asked if I had plans for a second book, I told her the only book that interested me was a sequel to the first. Rather than writing a huge scientific resource that was only interesting to the people who love extra nerdy details, I wanted to make this information more accessible to a wider audience. I wanted to provide people like you with the kind of practical help and advice that I could give you if we worked together in person. Without the belief she had in me, this follow-up book would not exist. She and the whole team at Octopus have been amazing at sharing my vision and bringing it to fruition.

Although I am the only named author on the front of the two books, I definitely do not deserve all the credit. Thank you to my wife, Sohee Carpenter, for being the first person ever to make me feel like I deserved to be ambitious with my career. Thank you to Luke Betts for believing in me so much that I rolled the dice and gambled on myself. Thank you to the wonderful team at Octopus, for helping me publish and elevate this book you are reading right now.

Last but not least, thank you to all of you who have supported me and cheered for me on social media over the years. Without you, none of this would be possible. You have helped change my life in more ways than I could ever put into words. I hope you can tell how much effort I have put into writing these books—I want to make you proud for granting me this opportunity in the first place.

# Image Credits

# About the Author

Ben Carpenter is a fitness coach and trusted source of no bullshit fat loss information who has spent his entire adult life working in the fitness industry, researching the real science and studies behind fat loss and answering questions with simplified, unbiased answers. Ben is a self-confessed "research nerd." As a personal trainer who is devoted to helping his clients and social media followers get the best results possible, his work isn't just about being up to date on the latest scientific research, but actually helping people put this information into practice. Ben was born in the UK but now lives in California with his wife.

- @bdccarpenter
- @bdccarpenter
- bencarpenter
- bencarpenterpersonaltraining